I0464809

THE
GEMS

THE
GEMS

The Guide for Effective Medical Students

HUSSAIN ISMA'EEL, MD

Copyright © 2015 by Hussain Isma'eel, MD.

Library of Congress Control Number:		2015901117
ISBN:	Hardcover	978-1-5035-3775-0
	Softcover	978-1-5035-3776-7
	eBook	978-1-5035-3772-9

All rights reserved. No part of this book may be reproduced or transmitted in any form or by any means, electronic or mechanical, including photocopying, recording, or by any information storage and retrieval system, without permission in writing from the copyright owner.

Any people depicted in stock imagery provided by Thinkstock are models, and such images are being used for illustrative purposes only.
Certain stock imagery © Thinkstock.

Print information available on the last page.

Rev. date: 02/13/2015

To order additional copies of this book, contact:
Xlibris
1-888-795-4274
www.Xlibris.com
Orders@Xlibris.com
635562

I am particularly privileged to introduce *"GEMS: The Guide for Effective Medical Students"* by Hussain Isma'eel and colleagues. I have spent the last 40 years of my life in Medicine, and the last fifteen in leadership positions in Medical Education. Prior to that, I had interacted with and taught numerous medical students at Harvard, Vanderbilt, and Emory universities' faculties of medicine. Having dealt with the challenges faced by medical students over the years, and the additional challenges faced by medical educators as the entire edifice of medical education was transformed radically over the past two decades, I can state with confidence that this "Guide" by Dr. Isma'eel and colleagues will be an invaluable tool.

In 2001, while Chair of the Department of Internal Medicine at the American University of Beirut, I first met and started to know Hussain Isma'eel as a resident physician. We then collaborated together after his return from Los Angeles during my tenure as Founding Dean of a new medical school at Lebanese American University, and now we have been working together again for the past 5 years in the Vascular Medicine Program at AUB. I am therefore thoroughly familiar with his superior talents and capacities as a thinker and a scientist, as well as an investigative physician. When he turned his attention to the education of medical students, I was therefore certain that he will have an effective impact. I was also certain his contribution will be based on a novel outlook, and presented with extreme logic and ease of understanding. This is exactly what students will find in this Guide. The result of Hussain deploying his considerable intellectual prowess in the service of helping medical students on their arduous journey is amply demonstrated in this Guide.

In addition to my admiration for his intellect as a thinker and scientist, I also had the privilege of sharing with Hussain many hours of discussion and analysis covering a wide range of personal, social,

5

political, and spiritual issues. Husain's clear and deeply held beliefs, and his understanding of the ultimate issues of life and death, are an integral part of all he does and writes. This book is no exception. Here, the students will learn of the writer's personality and his beliefs and ideas through the numerous reflective passages, which often introduce or conclude chapters relating to particular clinical skills or pearls of medical student learning. That he has chosen the heart as the central organ of demonstration for the skills being taught is emphatically reflective of the author's intention not only to edify the mind and improve physical skills in medicine, but also to penetrate the reader's "heart" and ask it to participate in reflecting on the deeper issues of life and death which medical students share with rest of humanity, but ever more acutely.

The aim of this work is to help the medical students be more of a healer. It accomplishes its purpose masterfully by teaching methodically and compassionately that true healing is a healing of the heart.

Kamal F Badr, MD, ASCI, AAP
Professor of Medicine (Nephrology and Hypertension)
Associate Dean for Medical Education, Faculty of Medicine
Director, Vascular Medicine Program
American University of Beirut, Beirut, Lebanon
Professor of Medicine (Adj.), Johns Hopkins University, Baltimore, MD, USA

This book is not about being a regular medical doctor, but about being a healer, with emphasis on how to become one. The background of this book is the belief in our responsibility to share with students of medicine, like myself, a practical guide delineating how a patient should be approached.

In stating that we are approaching the patient, we are stressing that each patient is unique and is a deciding entity. Only by holding the latter belief will we ensure that our thinking pyramid permits us to achieve a correct and comprehensive attitude toward the patient. This attitude in turn dictates behaviors that are projected in an aligned discipline. The core of this book is to provide the handy and simplified discipline that connects our belief, attitude, and behavior with the patient to address the patient's needs and last with, God willing, the favorable outcome we all desire all in the shortest line. This line is the line of the healers. In doing so, we should not disregard facts that are apparent to us out of personal agendas nor permit a false detail to steer us away from correctly identifying patterns of healing. Otherwise, we may go astray and take a different line than the one described above.

The goal of this guide is to provide recommendations that can be extrapolated to medicine in general, but with focus on the field of adult cardiology. To further clarify, out of practicality and my own limitations, kindly take note of the following:

1. The details that will be mentioned will change in time with more data and analytical power. Thus, please excuse our lack of foresight and assume the responsibility of updating these details yourself.
2. All the examples will be in the field of adult cardiology since this is our field (with some exceptions for analogy purposes).

3. The mechanisms that will be presented are in no way presented as perfect. Hence, any feedback is more than welcome for us to learn and refine our own personal approach.
4. The end goal is to promote health through combating humanity's enemy: our ignorance and that of others.
5. This book is intended to serve in the name of the Merciful and may he be our evident guide.

Acknowledgments

While writing this, a group of medical students corroborated this guide. To Bader Kfoury, Lara Hilal, Petra Chamseddine, Rami Diab, and Hassan Doumiati, I am forever grateful. My colleague and friend Dr. Fouad Boulos and Mr. Mohammad Ali Al Masri contributed to the figures.

Furthermore, as a visiting scholar to the Cleveland Clinic Cardiology Department, I saw how they lead by example, hence verifying this guide.

Last, enduring life in general required the support of my parents (Ali and Souheila), my brother (Hassan), sisters (Nihal, Noor and Dana), brother-in-law (Nasseem), a number of friends (Ghassan Hamadeh, Jaafar Makki, Namir Damluji and Abbas Makki), and my love Zahraa. I am blessed by the Almighty to have you all; his kindness permitted this experience to become a reality.

Contributing Authors

Wissam Alajaji, MD
Resident Internal Medicine
Case Western Reserve University

Imad Elhajj, PhD
Associate Professor
Department of Electrical and Computer Engineering
American University of Beirut

Mohammad ElOubeidi, MD, MPH
Professor of Medicine
Associate Chair, Department of Internal Medicine
American University of Beirut Medical Center

Fatima Ghaddar, MD, MPH candidate
Faculty of Health Sciences
American University of Beirut

Wael Jaber, MD
Head Center for Advanced Ischemic Heart Disease
Medical Director of the Cardiovascular Imaging Core Laboratory
Cleveland Clinic

Hani Tamim, PhD
Associate Professor, Department of Internal Medicine
Director, Biostatistics Unit, Clinical Research Institute
American University of Beirut Medical Center

Oussama Wazni, MD
Director of the Outpatient Electrophysiology Department
Codirector of the Ventricular Arrhythmia Center
Cleveland Clinic

Code of the Discipline

1. The Healer is You
   A. Pattern Recognition: From Complaint to Differential Diagnosis Formation
   B. Prime Statistics: Understanding the Power of a Tool
   C. Personal Code is Self-Knowledge

2. Outcome-Based Healing Approach: From Prophecy to Artificial Intelligence
3. Healing INDEX: Our Unified Tool in Practicing Patient Healing
   I. I - Intensity
   II. N - Navigation
   III. D - Develop plan jointly
   IV. E - Expectations to be set
   V. X - eXtras that need to be dealt with

4. The Universal Common Source of the Four Principles of Medical Ethics in Application
5. Choosing Your Specialty: A Set of Questions and FACTS
6. Healing: Success is from Within to Climate Creation
7. Literature in Medical Education: Living Multiple Lives

Accompanying each chapter is a fable for personal reflection. This was included to permit some extrapolation of some of the presented concepts into the realm of self-development.

The Healer Is You

To start this book, we first define our role, and that role is that of the healer. The healer's role emanates from the belief that we are healers, which will lead to developing the commensurate attitude and subsequently project a set of behaviors. Of the several behaviors that need to be adopted, we need to highlight a major one, which is knowledge seeking. This knowledge starts with knowledge of one's self and thereafter progresses outward. With this understanding, healers acknowledge that humans are complete entities both physical and emotional—equal to themselves—and therefore approach them as such. Following increasing knowledge is increasing responsibility to be proactive and to heal.

In ancient Semite languages, to heal referred to relieving the human from a disturbing force that is altering his course of living. Naturally, before science developed, humans used to bring in the mystical components into the picture. Hence, the human was God's creature to build the world, the disturbing force touching the human is Satanic— the enemy—and therefore the relief would come from aligning with God to combat this force.

In some metaphors, the human is portrayed as living in this life— referred to as a maze or the "liver"— continuously combating difficulties and avoiding getting lost. The reason the liver was chosen is because anatomically speaking, the liver has sinusoidal tracts that takes in unclean blood and detoxifies it to permit the exit of clean blood. The liver is also referred to as "the black" in some cultures. Therefore, the human is to live in "the liver" and work his way through the difficulties he faces guided by the light of divinity to enlighten his path in the black, undergoing detoxification and emerging pure and clean. This is the journey, and healers are prescribers of light to the troubled.

The above can be summarized as follows: Humans are created in a liver—the black—and when they patiently fight through (both internally themselves and externally), they are gifted by his light.

Accordingly, healers in the old tradition were portrayed as individuals who would listen, examine, diagnose, and intervene. Along with that understanding, on one hand, old stories showed wizards and witches hitting individuals to drive out evil spirits. On the other hand and at a different level and scale, prophets were shown to heal humans by ordering evil spirits to leave the "toxified" human. In the former situation, hitting served as the intervention, whereas in the latter situation, ordering and the use of verbal commands served as the intervention.

Later on in history, science started to enter the picture and all the mystical ideas were further pushed away. Accordingly, instead of attributing illness to the touch of evil, humans started understanding the impact of our predispositions and family history or genetics; the impact of environmental forces or epigenetics; and the impact of dietary intake, unhealthy lifestyle habits, and autoimmune disorders. Interestingly, when science is unable to explain a disease, i.e., the cause that secondarily leads to the disease is unknown, we refer to the disease as primary, i.e., idiopathic, which is synonymous to the unknown in the old tradition. Given that God is the biggest unknown in the old tradition; this led some contemporary cultures to misunderstand this primary as The Primary. This understanding is wrong because we should not blame science's limitations today on the Healer. It is our duty to acknowledge; what we do not know today will be uncovered tomorrow by science. The Primary is innocent from being the cause of disease, *regardless of whether we believe in The Primary or not* (and I believe). The principle is that no disease is primary, and there is always a cause; and this cause is waiting to be uncovered by scientists.

No proof for the above principle is clearer than psychiatric diseases that are now treatable either by cognitive behavioral therapy, in which verbal approaches are the intervention, or by electroconvulsive therapy, which is equivalent to being hit. No proof of the above principle is clearer than the significantly witnessed prolongation in human survival, which doubled in the last century or so. Therefore, if we scientists accept that the false understanding of the concept of the primary prevails, then we allow false ideas to take root, and such false ideas can affect people's belief in us. In doing so, we allow doubt to prevail over trust in the relationship between healers and their patients.

Similarly, in a higher dimension, should people's belief in us—the healers—be shaken, then this will affect the whole profession at large. This will result in people going back to the mystics, and these today have different names and sell their products under different brands, even in supermarkets, and with no evidence whatsoever. Unfortunately, euphemisms have permitted these to be called natural medicine. These euphemisms indicate that what we provide is not natural. The truth is that what we provide is *the* natural medicine; our medicine is the product of the sound experimental methods of natural sciences. We should not permit anything that allows people lose trust in us. If we do so, then people will have less commitment to science, to accepting science as the path toward treating disease in this world, and to donate to scientific institutions to further invest in scientific discoveries. This also results in people's reduced adherence to therapies and less understanding and acceptance of our limitations, and lowers our self-respect and therefore others' respect for us, thus leading to anger and demotivation. Healing is not a ten-minute one-stop-and-shop visit. Healing involves following a process in a path with tremendous responsibilities and ramifications.

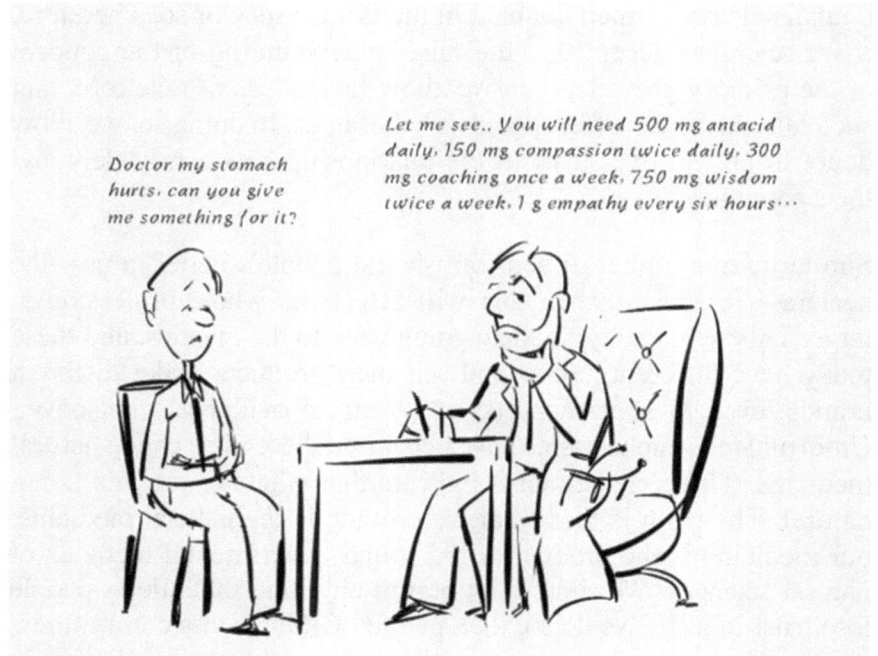

Illustration drawn by Dr. Fouad Boulos

It is our responsibility as healers to combat the above situation, and this can be achieved through patient-centered care. Patient-centered care involves the following process: listening, inquiring, examining, requesting tests for more data, analyzing, recognizing a pattern, formulating a plan, being transparent, empowering the patient for joint decisions, remembering that you are the expert and the coach, not being defensive nor offensive, intervening, measuring response, revisiting the approach, being the custodian of the patient's best interests, ensuring the patient's satisfaction, attending to the patient's needs (from the most intimate to the most distant), and showing the patient and his family that you are a caring and loving person. The above process ensures that healing is bound to be achieved, even if the patient dies, for you have become the healer. Healers carry the lanterns of science in this life and practice with knowledge, empathy, experience, wisdom, kindness, firmness, and compassion. This is our systematic approach.

From Differential Diagnosis Formation to Pattern Recognition and Disease Identification

During the theoretical knowledge acquisition years, we were taught by being provided a "title," which is the name of the disease. Then, we were taught the symptoms and signs (these along with test results will be referred to as "disease features" later). Afterwards, we were taught how to treat the disease and the course of healing. During the clinical years, we are supposed to learn how to gather information about the disease (the symptoms and signs), then group these pieces of information under a differential or a set of diseases that causes such findings, then subject the patient to tests to narrow down the differential and identify the disease, then provide the treatment and observe the course of healing. We note that we start with knowing the disease and then describing its features (the pattern it presents) in the theory learning years, then we work to identify the disease from the features during the clinical years. The latter is pattern recognition and is what we do in clinical practice.

Theoretical Years Knowledge Acquisition Process

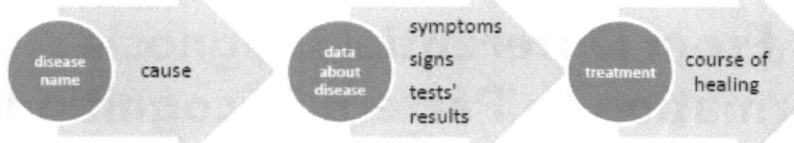

Clinical Years Differential Diagnosis Formation Process

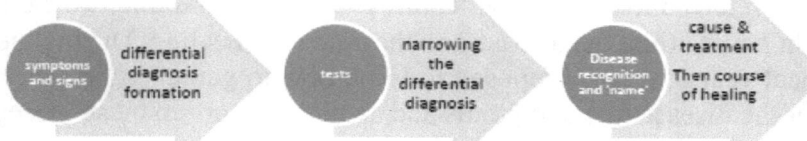

Naturally, since what we are performing in the clinical years is like a backward "walk" relative to the theory learning years, it is absolutely normal to feel uneasy at the beginning. This chapter aims to coach us on how to "walk backwards" and hopefully alleviate this uneasiness. To achieve that, we present Figure 2 below. The starting point is when the patient informs us of the reason behind the visit, i.e., the chief complaint. As soon as the patient provides us with that piece of information, we form three prominent pillars that carry the platform from which we will launch our probing pathway. These three pillars are

1. The patient's gender
2. The patient's age
3. The organ/system dysfunction that can be causing this chief complaint

With these three pillars, we are supposed to examine all our existing theoretical knowledge and start shuffling things to determine the possibilities that can cause this chief complaint, while taking into consideration epidemiological information related to age and gender.

To clarify, while intussusception occurs in infants, it is very rare in adults. Therefore, we will not be thinking of intussusception as a cause of abdominal pain in a 55-year-old gentleman. The same applies to diseases that are more likely to occur in one gender than the other. However, this is certainly less prominent than the age factor. It is worth noting that sexual organ-related diseases are always something we should be thinking of and naturally impacts the probability of occurrence of certain diseases. *In brief, with every piece of information we add to the chief complaint, the probability of certain diseases is either increasing or decreasing.*

To make this more interactive, we take the case of a 25-year-old lady who is experiencing palpitations.

As expected, the minute palpitations and the age and gender are mentioned. We then open the differential list on the right-hand corner of Figure 2.

We then move to ask generic questions that are applicable to most, if not all, complaints, such as

1. When was the first time you felt this complaint?
2. When was the last time it happened?
3. How long does it last?

More focused questions pertaining to palpitations can then be asked, such as

1. Are the palpitations regular or irregular?
2. Are the palpitations fast or slow?
3. Do they wake you up from sleep, or do they happen only during the day?

At this stage, we are ready to ask more questions that are related to the primary organ that we think this complaint is attributed to, which is the heart. *However, given that the complaint is an electrical function complaint, then we are supposed to ask arrhythmia questions first followed by pump and angina questions.* Had the complaint been shortness of breath or lower extremity edema, then we would have started with the pump function-related questions.

Upon completing the questions pertaining to the primary organ of suspicion, we move to questions about the other organs/systems, or secondary organs, under which the diseases in our differential fall. Hyperthyroidism is among the common causes of palpitation. Thus, we should ask endocrine-related questions, starting with those pertaining to hyperthyroidism followed by those that are related to other etiologies such as pheochromocytoma.

Subsequently, we move from one organ/system to another depending on the etiologies we listed in the differential until we have covered them all until step 5 or 6. Ideally, the differential list should be arranged from the most possible to the least possible based on the age and gender of the patient. This is not a must at this stage.

Figure 2. Stepwise approach to a case of palpitations

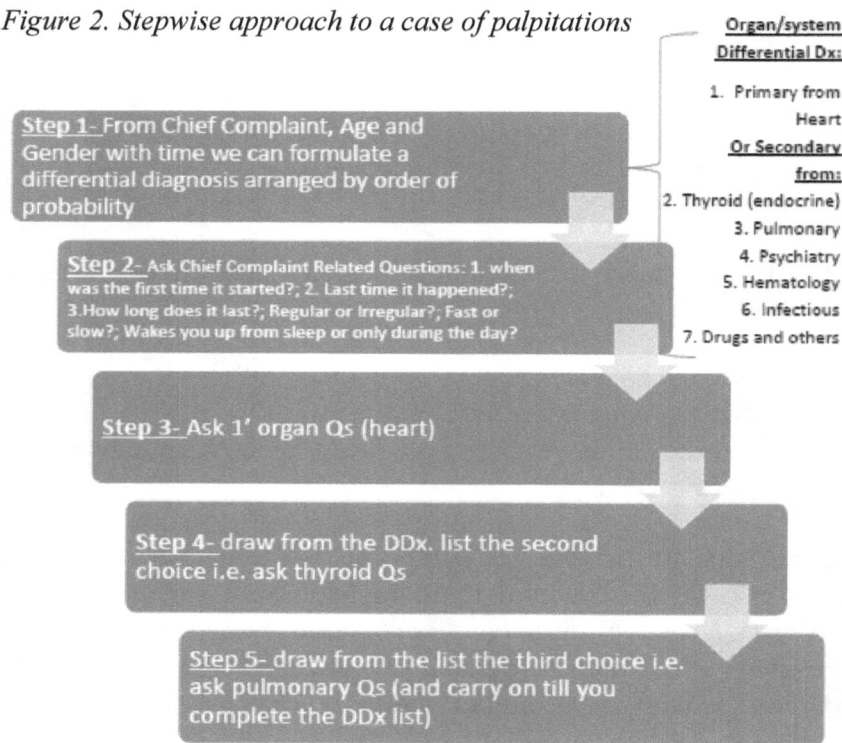

Organ/system
Differential Dx:

1. Primary from Heart
Or Secondary from:
2. Thyroid (endocrine)
3. Pulmonary
4. Psychiatry
5. Hematology
6. Infectious
7. Drugs and others

Step 1- From Chief Complaint, Age and Gender with time we can formulate a differential diagnosis arranged by order of probability

Step 2- Ask Chief Complaint Related Questions: 1. when was the first time it started?; 2. Last time it happened?; 3.How long does it last?; Regular or Irregular?; Fast or slow?; Wakes you up from sleep or only during the day?

Step 3- Ask 1' organ Qs (heart)

Step 4- draw from the DDx. list the second choice i.e. ask thyroid Qs

Step 5- draw from the list the third choice i.e. ask pulmonary Qs (and carry on till you complete the DDx list)

It is important that we move in this process in an organized and systematic manner to ensure the following outcomes:

1. This will help us sort our thinking process before moving to the next step, which is the physical exam, so we actually focus that on the organ under suspicion.
2. This is how we will be writing our medical note, i.e., in a stepwise manner of documenting the patient's responses to an organ/system questioning approach, which indicates that we were systematic in our probing.
3. This will ensure comprehensiveness so we do not overlook some possibilities.

After completing all the steps detailed in Figure 2, we move to acquiring the information needed to have a more comprehensive understanding of the patient (Figure 3). This approach is similar to the flow described in the INDEX chapter with the iAMOSMS acronym, and we will not dwell more on this here. Thereafter, we are ready to proceed with the physical exam.

1' Organ (heart) Related Questions:

1. Arrhythmia focused (syncope, dizziness, family history of arrhythmia or sudden death)
2. General Cardio Questions: Chest pain, shortness of breath, diaphoresis, decreased exercise tolerance, PND, orthopnea, lower extremity edema

2' Organ oriented Questions:

1. Thyroid and endocrine questions
2. Psychiatry (anxiety)
3. Pulmonary
4. Hematology (anemia)
5. Infectious
6. Drugs and others

System/Morbidities/Medications Questions:

1. Complete Review of Systems
2. Get all Drugs/Allergies and Travel History

Support System Questions:

1. Where does the patient live?
2. And how far is this from where the work up is going to be carried?
3. Is the patient dependent on others for transportation?
4. What insurance coverage the patient has? Possibly none.
5. Will there be any financial challenges that prohibit performing any of the tests?

Your aim from the Support System Question section is to identify any challenges that can stop the patient from seeking care. So be caring, inquisitive and resourceful to offer solutions.

I
Am
O

S
M

S

Perform Physical Exam also 1' Organ Oriented then Systemic Oriented

At this point, we are supposed to have determined which of the etiologies' features the patient confirmed and which ones were dismissed by the patient.

Then, we move on to synthesis, which is the step that takes us beyond data collection.

Synthesis is the end result of the dialectic you are having with yourself: Does the patient have this disease or not? It is basically the question you ask yourself when you pause for a split second between listening to the patient and listening to your inner voice. Many times, this is followed by the next question: Have I missed anything? If you missed an etiology, then you ask the questions about this etiology. To synthesize, we take all the pieces into the analytic department in our head to RECOGNIZE THE PATTERN (Figure 4). Essentially we are performing disease identification through a probability-based stepwise approach:

1. The more features of a disease the patient has confirmed, the more likely that the patient has this disease.
2. The fewer features of a disease the patient has displayed, the less likely it is that the patient has this disease. (This rule is not always true, but is the case in most situations.)
3. Should a feature that is very specific to a certain etiology appear, then this directly increases the probability that this is the cause of the complaint. For example, the presence of irregular heartbeats or history of sudden death in the family significantly increases the probability of arrhythmia. More importantly, even if the arrhythmia is not the cause, given the gravity of the consequences of missing an arrhythmia in a person with a family history of sudden death, we have to keep arrhythmias on our differential and work up the patient for this. This similarly applies also to having a history of peptic ulcer disease, which suggests that there may be underlying anemia.
4. *Apply the principle "Common things remain common."* Out of all the cases of palpitations we will encounter in our career, <1% will be pheochromocytoma because of the rarity of the entity. Thus, even if the patient meets several criteria that fit pheochromocytoma, which therefore increases the likelihood of having pheochromocytoma by 10 times, the end probability of pheochromocytoma will still be <10%.
5. In the elderly and those with multiple comorbidities, more than one disease leading to the chief complaint can be present simultaneously, whereas in relatively young and healthy individuals, only one disease is probably the cause of the chief complaint.

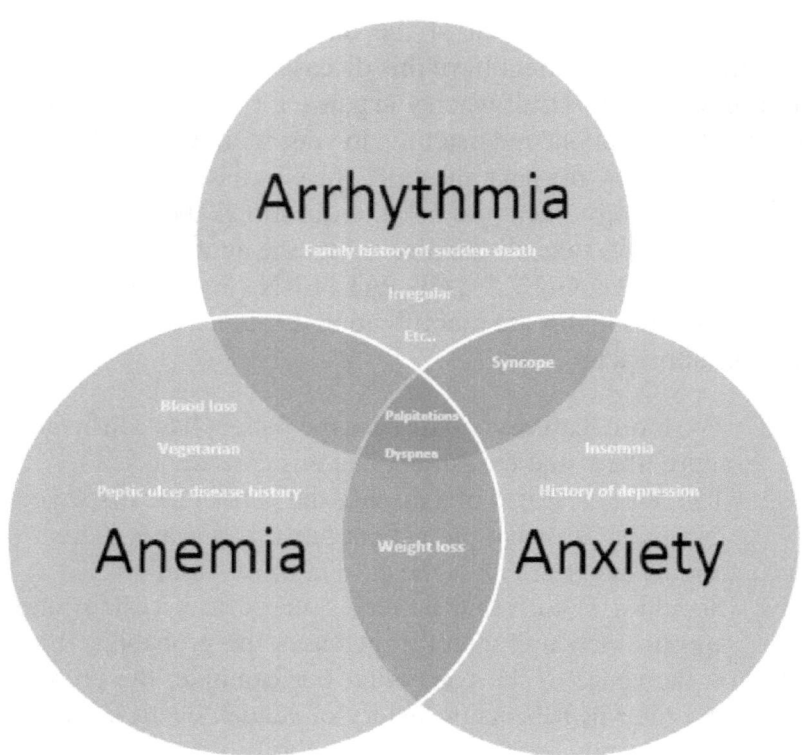

As we all see from Figure 4, the chief complaint, i.e., palpitations, is present in the overlapping area of all three etiologies. However, we can distinguish the etiologies from one another from the data collected from our history taking and physical exam steps.

Collecting the features highlighted in bold yellow above in a systematic manner ensures that we have a clear thought process that pays off in the management of our patients.

By applying the five synthesis principles, above we are supposed to arrange the differential in a descending order of probability. This in turn should be reflected when we write our medical note.

Consider the following:

Ms. XY is a 25-year-old lady experiencing palpitations with features in favor of hyperthyroidism, for example, as the underlying cause, some features of anxiety, but no features of valve disease, no features of an underlying arrhythmia or of a febrile illness, etc.

If we expand the above couple of sentences by replacing each etiology with the symptoms of each etiology, we will have the section of the history of presenting illness in our note. In reverse, the end result of synthesis is the three sentences above. How close our synthesis is to the truth is how powerful we are as disease-identifying physicians. This is one of our important powers as clinicians, and it grows with practice, reading, commitment, and experience. To further train ourselves in pattern recognition, let us perform Exercises 1, 2 and 3 below.

Exercise 1: Match the following symptoms with the corresponding heart dysfunction by inserting near the symptom the number corresponding to the heart dysfunction that can cause it (each symptom may be caused by more than one dysfunction, but always arrange them starting with the most likely).

Symptom	Heart Dysfunction
extremity edema	1. Heart pump dysfunction (heart failure or valve dysfunction)
Chest pain at rest	
Fast heartbeats	
Syncope	2. Coronary disease (atherosclerosis or Prinzmetal)
Increased abdominal girth	
Orthopnea	
Chest pain with exertion	3. Lower Electrical abnormality
Dyspnea at rest	
Dyspnea with exertion	

Irregular heartbeats

From Exercise 1, we should further appreciate the symptoms associated with the three major groups of heart dysfunction: electrical, pump, and coronary abnormality-related dysfunctions.

Exercise 2a: Arrange the symptoms below in the circles of etiologies that they may be part of.

- nervousness about the possibility of losing control and doing something embarrassing;
- fear of dying
- coughing up blood
- irregular heartbeat
- terror; a sense that something unimaginably horrible is about to occur and that one is powerless to prevent it;
- a need to escape
- anxiety
- sweating
- shortness of breath
- dizziness
- squeezing or sharp chest pains
- pain that radiates to extremities and/or back
- difficulty breathing; a sense of feeling smothered
- tingling or numbness in the hands
- nausea
- coughing
- unexplained fatigue
- stomach upset
- dizziness, lightheadedness, nausea
- hot flashes or chills
- trembling and shaking
- dreamlike sensations or perceptual distortions

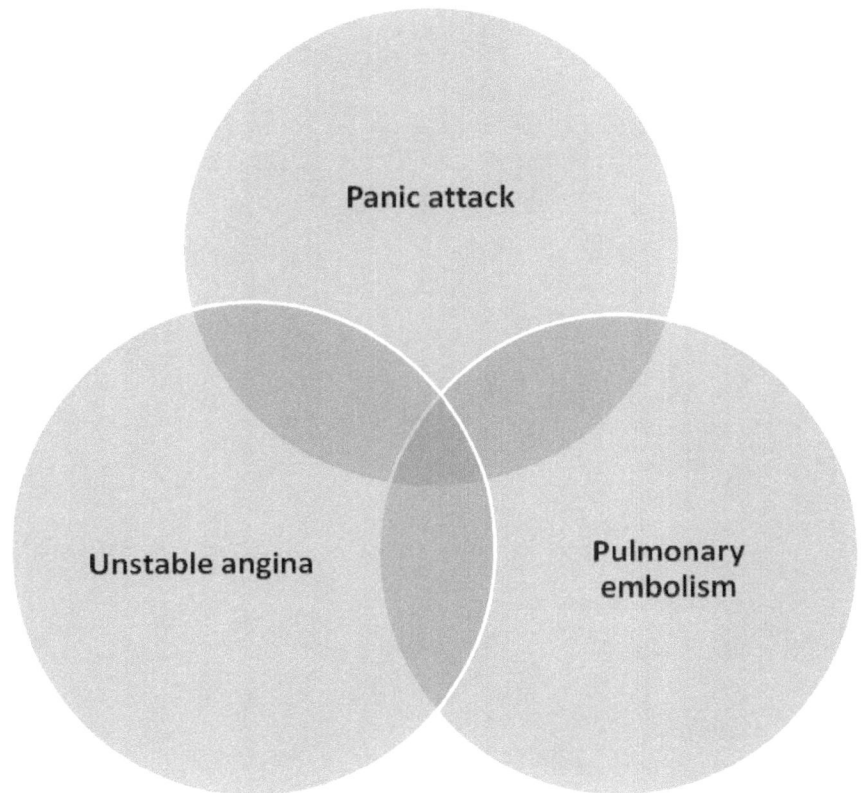

Exercise 2b: Arrange the symptoms below in the circles of etiologies that they may be part of.

- use of laxatives
- heartburn
- diarrhea
- constipation
- clay-colored stools
- melena
- hematemesis
- jaundice
- food intolerance
- indigestion
- history of gallbladder disease
- use of antacids
- nausea
- vomiting
- dark urine
- family history of GI malignancy
- dysphagia

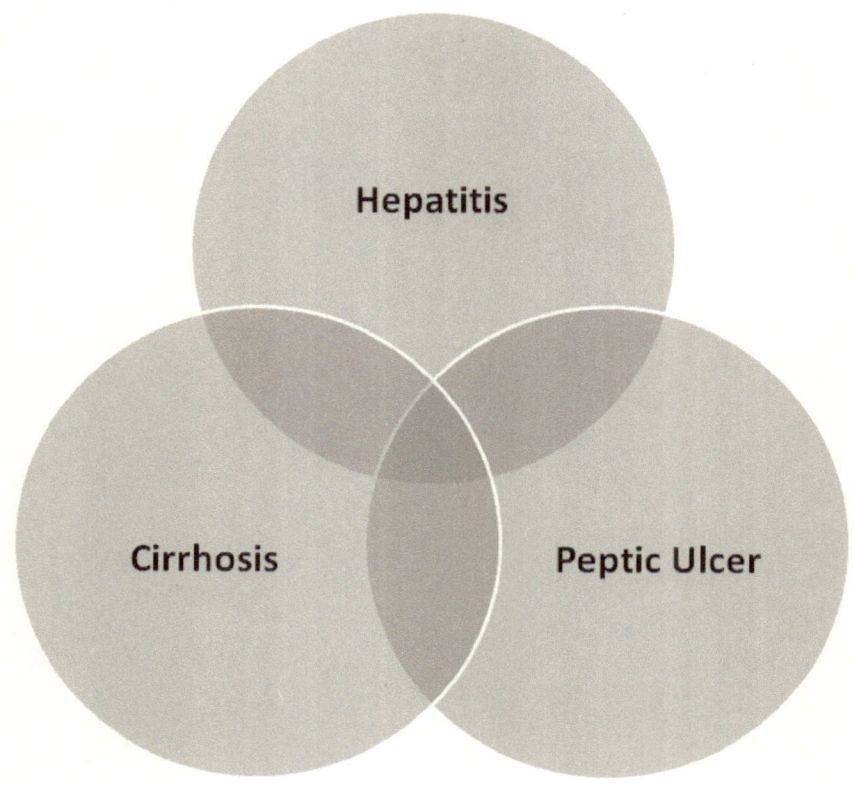

From Exercise 2, we should have recognized several points.

1. There is a significant overlap between etiologies.
2. When such a significant overlap between etiologies occurs, more features are needed to further perform the separation needed for pattern recognition. This may be achieved if there is a history of myocardial infarction, if the person is a 20-year-old, or if the person has a history of recurrent deep venous thrombosis.
3. In the absence of "strong" features such as those described above, features that are the results of tests become a must to properly perform the differentiation.
4. Given that the area of overlap is significant between a relatively non–life-threatening condition, which is a panic attack, and two other very lethal conditions if missed (pulmonary embolism and unstable angina), we must be very considerate

to the lethal conditions and not be inclined to underappreciate the patient's complaints and dismiss them as a panic attack.

5. How to properly balance between our duty to rule out lethal conditions and also remain cost conscious is a challenge by itself that we learn in due time and has its own pathways.

Exercise 3: Expand the following statements by replacing the diseases with symptoms and signs from the lists above.

1. Ms. UA is a 55-year-old lady who presented to the emergency department with symptoms and signs suggestive of unstable angina and, to a lesser degree, suggestive of pulmonary embolism or a panic attack.
2. Mr. LC is a 60-year-old gentleman known to be an alcoholic who presented to the emergency department with symptoms and signs suggestive of liver cirrhosis and, to a lesser degree, of esophageal varicosities complicating this cirrhosis. He is fairly unlikely to have hepatitis or peptic ulcer disease.

Upon completing this exercise, we should have recognized what is it that we are doing when we reduce the symptoms and signs to the short statements above, i.e., synthesis through pattern recognition by probing and applying the probability-based stepwise approach of the five principles above.

Understanding the power of a tool

Hani Tamim and Hussain Isma'eel

In medical school, they teach us about the sensitivity, specificity and other features of an investigational tool. However, like most of this book's chapters, in our practice, we emphasize the message we can deliver to the patient after subjecting the patient to the test. We are outcome driven. Hence, what we want you to embrace is the understanding of the power of the tool. By this, we mean, how can the answers we get from the tool shift a diagnosis upward or downward on the probability scale? The inherent significance of this understanding will reflect where it is most needed: linking our understanding to our communication with the patient. Furthermore, since we are underscoring "the power of the tool," this power needs to be independent of the patients' characteristics as much as possible. It should be a tool function, not a patient function, and it should not vary with the prevalence of disease in various populations.

Other factors may favor one tool more than another, such as accessibility, cost, and user friendliness. But for the purpose of this chapter, we will focus on the above factors only. This chapter aims to thoroughly explain the integration of using likelihood ratios to form the messages to be delivered to the patient and in walking through the scheme below.

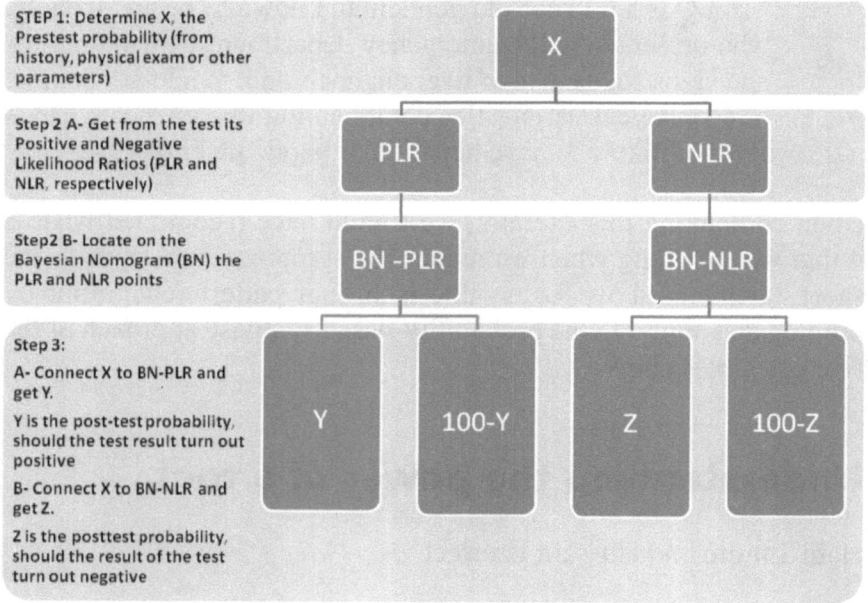

The patient is mostly interested in knowing X (pretest probability), and Y (posttest probability, if the result of test suggests that the disease is present) or Z (posttest probability if the result of the test suggests that the disease is not present).

The patient does not want to know about sensitivities and specificities of the test.

The patient should not be given affirmative 0% or 100% answers; this is not only false but can also break the trust bond.

To determine what is Y and what is Z we need to use the Bayesian Nomogram (see below). How we do this and the benefits will be explained in the context of a case of a patient presenting to

Let us start from the point where we have formulated a differential diagnosis and we have arranged the etiologies by descending order of probability. Doing so, we have mentally assigned for each etiology a quantitative percentage that the patient has it. This was achieved using the history and the physical exam only. *Since this probability is set before subjecting the patient to the tool (the test), it is referred to as the pretest probability. Ideally, if we include all the possible etiologies in the differential list, then the sum of the probabilities of all the etiologies should reach 100%. Subsequently, we should find the true cause of the disease in the list—and maybe more than one etiology are interplaying.*

The power of the tool, as alluded to earlier, in our understanding is its likelihood ratios. More clearly, what we need to conclude after the test and relay to the patient is

1- If the test result turns out to be positive (disease is likely present), how much is the probability of the patient having the disease? Or,

2- If the test's result turns out to be negative (disease is likely absent), how much is the probability that the patient still has the disease?

After the patient is subjected to the test, there are two routes: either the test favors the presence of the disease or disfavors it. It is fundamental here to remind ourselves that we are dealing with probabilities, and in this domain, there is no 0% or 100%. The outcome is not binary [0 (no disease) or 1 (disease is present)].

The probability of the disease after the test result comes out is the posttest probability.

From a pretest probability of X, we move on to a posttest probability Y where Y > X if the result favors the disease or to Z where Z < X if the result disfavors the presence of the disease. *Y is not 100%, and Z is not 0%.* (Before proceeding any further, we want to highlight that how X is calculated is part of the pattern recognition chapter where this will be further explained.)

Again, being patient centered, we should remember that the patient wants to know the following:

1. What is the pretest probability of disease from the history and physical exam?
2. What is the posttest probability of disease after the test result comes out?

These are the two central questions that need to be answered. After answering these, management issues are to be discussed, and the theme in the INDEX chapter is followed.

One of the core messages in this chapter is that patients may not understand sensitivity or specificity, and we should not expect them to do so. However, in common language, the patients do understand how likely it is that they have or do not have the disease. These are lay terms; remember that it is our responsibility to ensure our message is delivered. We are responsible for what we say. Some patients may not even want a number but might request a qualitative categorization, such as low, intermediate, or highly likely to have or have not a disease. In some cases, such as the one discussed below, this can be provided; however, this is not true in all situations. Of note, the gravitational pull behind this conversation from the patients' side is the patients' desire to reach certainty, i.e., the binary outcome: have (100%) or not have (0%) the disease. This is a commonly requested term, the bottom line, which we should resist providing at every cost because this is not only untrue and contradicts the science, but also can lead to more deleterious outcomes. One of the undesired outcomes is trust-bond breaking should the final result contradict a result that was communicated earlier based on a single test. Be empathic, and note that the patients' feelings are not to be toyed with. Thus, stay objective and scientific, and avoid impulsive drives in the conversation to be affirmative. This affirmation can harm you and the patient, even if your intentions were good, such as trying to appease the patient's anxiety. Be both kind and firm, and build/ preserve the trust bond.

The 2X2 table below clearly explains how the sensitivity, specificity, and positive likelihood ratio (PLR) and negative likelihood ratio (NLR) are derived. We promote focusing on likelihood ratios and in particular on memorizing this understanding:

The PLR is the probability of a positive test in those with disease/ probability of positive test in those without disease.

The NLR is the probability of a negative test in those with disease/ probability of negative test in those without disease.

The above two statements are important to memorize because they clearly state what we sometimes forget: *Our tools are not 100% accurate. Hence, even if a test result suggests that a disease is present, always keep in mind that the disease might not be present; the converse is also true.*

To determine what Y is and what Z is, we need to use the Bayesian nomogram (see below). How we do this and the benefits will be explained in the context of a case of a patient presenting to rule out coronary artery disease.

Estimating the sensitivity and specificity of diagnostic test

True diagnosis
'gold standard'

<table>
<tr><th></th><th></th><th>Disease present</th><th>Disease absent</th><th></th></tr>
<tr><td rowspan="4">Test Results</td><td>Positive</td><td>a

True positive</td><td>b

False positive</td><td>a + b</td></tr>
<tr><td>Negative</td><td>c

False negative</td><td>d

True negative</td><td>c + d</td></tr>
<tr><td></td><td>a + c</td><td>b + d</td><td></td></tr>
</table>

Sensitivity=a/(a+c)
Specificity=d/(b+d)

Positive predictive value=a/(a+b)
Negative predictive value=d/(c+d)

Positive
likelihood =   Probability of positive test in those with disease
ratio   Probability of positive test in those without disease

= TP rate/FP rate

= (a/[a+c]) / (b/[b+d])

= Sensitivity / (1-specificity)

Negative
likelihood =   Probability of negative test in those with disease
ratio   Probability of negative test in those without disease

= FN rate/TN rate

= (c/[a+c]) / (d/[b+d])

= (1-sensitivity) / specificity

Likelihood ratios have a number of useful properties:

- Because they are based on a ratio of sensitivity and specificity, they do no vary in different populations or settings.
- They can be used directly at the individual patient level.
- They allow the clinician to quantitate the probability of disease for any individual patient.

CASE: Mr. S.L. is a 65-year-old gentleman known to be hypertensive and is well controlled on medications, smoker (35 pack-years), and has LDL 136 mg/dl and HDL 31 mg/dl, who noted recently to have new onset chest pain, diffuse, upon exercise, and relieved by rest. His physician recommended a stress echocardiography to rule out obstructive coronary artery disease.

The Question: Does this patient have obstructive coronary artery disease (CAD)? What are the posttest probabilities of obstructive CAD based on the result of the stress echocardiography?

Step 1: Calculate the pretest probability of obstructive CAD "X" using history (and physical exam features in other cases).

X can be calculated using one of several models [Diamond Forrester (DF), updated DF, Morise model, Duke model, COROSCORE, or the NICE model]. For the sake of this case, we will use the updated DF model. To do that, we have to determine the type of angina we are discussing. First, answer the three questions in column A below, then based on column B, label the patient's angina.

Diamond Forrester Criteria for Angina Types

Column A	Column B
Ask 3 questions	Total the number of "yes" answers to identify symptom pattern
• Is chest pain substernal?	0 of 3=Asymptomatic
• Is chest pain brought on by exertion or stress?	1 of 3=Non-anginal chest pain
• Is chest pain relieved within 10 minutes by rest or NTG?	2 of 3=Atypical angina
	3 of 3=Typical angina

Answer to Step 1a: The patient turns out to have 2/3 and therefore has atypical angina.

From there, using the calculator in **Genders T S et al., Eur Heart J 2011; eurheartj.ehr014,** calculate the pretest probability. The pretest probability of having obstructive CAD (defined as >=50% stenosis on >=1 vessel in conventional angiography) is 54.2%. We can alternatively use the original Diamond Forrester method if we do not have access to the calculator.

Step 2

A. From the table below, we obtain the negative and positive likelihood ratios of the test we chose. For stress echocardiography, the PLR is 3.7, and the NLR is 0.19.

Likelihood ratios of various noninvasive tests

	Positive Likelihood Ratio	Negative Likelihood Ratio
Exercise ECG	1.79	0.68
Exercise SPECT	3.22	0.18
Stress Echo	3.70	0.19
Stress CMR	4.15	0.21
Cardiac CT	3.00	0.06

Then, use the Bayesian nomogram below, and on the vertical axis on the left, which denotes the pretest probability line, locate the 54.2% point.

B.

- To calculate the posttest probability if the stress echocardiography is positive, we locate on the likelihood ratios vertical axis the PLR point, which is 3.7. Connect the pretest probability point to the PLR point to form a line— *the solid black line*—that intersects the posttest probability vertical line on the right-hand side.

  The point of intersection is between 75% and 80%. This corresponds to the posttest probability of obstructive CAD should the stress echocardiography result turn out to be positive.

- To calculate the posttest probability if the stress echocardiography is negative, we locate on the likelihood ratios vertical axis the NLR point, which is 0.19. Connect the pretest probability point to the NLR point to form a line—*the dashed black line*—that intersects the posttest probability vertical line on the right corner.

The point of intersection is between 15% and 20%. This corresponds to the posttest probability of obstructive CAD should the stress echocardiography result turn out to be negative for obstructive CAD.

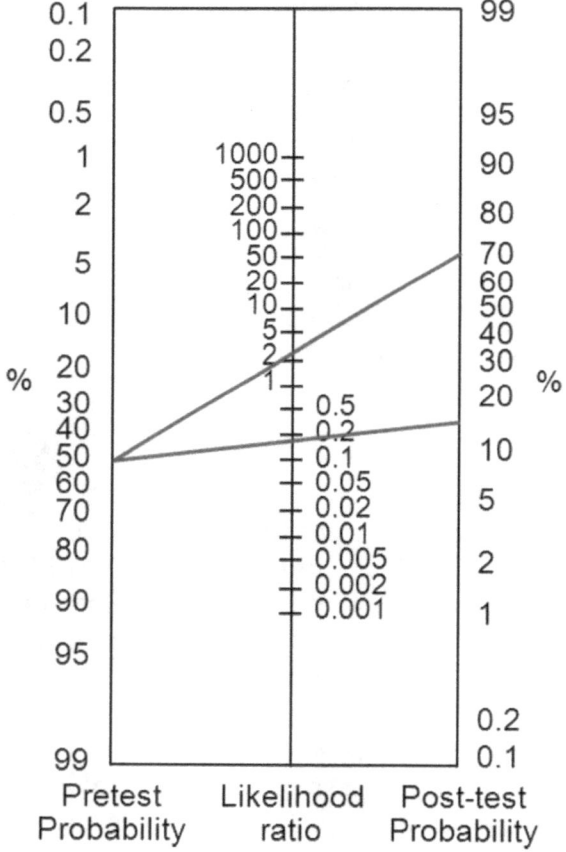

Thus, the patient's pretest probability was 54.2% for having obstructive CAD as per his history. Depending on the stress echocardiography result, his posttest probability will be either 75% to 80% (disease is present if the stress echocardiography is positive) or *15% to 20% (disease is also present if the stress echocardiography is negative)*.

At this point, we have reached the moment of truth: communicating the message.

With the above understanding, it should become clear to you that regardless of the result of the stress echocardiography, the possibility of having obstructive CAD is present. Therefore, cautiously selecting your words to match this understanding is the art that we hope you will master—and you can easily do so.

Visualize yourself sitting with Mr. SL. He has already undergone the stress echocardiography test and got back to you with the result.

Scenario A: The result is positive.

The objectives of the communication should be to

- Inform him of the posttest probability of having the disease, i.e., 75% to 80%
- Inform him that a cardiac catheterization is warranted
- Confirm that there is a 20% chance that he will not have disease

I: Your stress echo suggests that you have obstructive disease and a cardiac catheterization is warranted at this stage.

SL: Are we certain that I have obstructive disease?

I: There is a 15% to 20% chance that you do not, and this is what I wish for you, but we cannot tell before the cath.

SL: Is there any other option so I can avoid cardiac catheterization?

I: Cardiac catheterization is the reference standard, and at this stage, since the probability of disease is high and you have chest pain, then another test is not a good choice.

Scenario B: The result is negative.

I: Your stress echocardiography does not suggest that you have obstructive coronary disease, and further studies to investigate other causes are needed. We will also be providing you with preventive measures for coronary disease by optimizing your medications.

SL: Are we certain that I do not have obstructive disease?

I: There is a 15% to 20% that you do have obstructive coronary disease. But given that the results came out negative, we can give a trial of medical treatment and have you come back shortly to reassess your situation.

Personal Code is Self-Knowledge

In line with the principle set in the first paragraph—"to become, first know who you are"—this section is a reflection highlighting the importance of counting your blessings and knowing your limits, for it is within these two fine acts that you exist; forgetting your blessings might lead to unwarranted anger, which in turn spoils judgment. Conversely, overappreciation of these blessings may lead to self-conceit, i.e., you think you are not subject to questioning, and that thought therefore pushes you to cross your limits. Know that we are all subject to questioning, so stay within your limits. On the other hand, drawing tighter limits may reflect a lack of confidence, which is self-restrictive. Conversely, not drawing them may diffuse your efforts. Set your own limits before they are set for you, and be ready to grow smoothly knowing that early bloomers risk frostbite.

One of the hallmarks of social development and civilization building is respect for numbers. Numbers are key identifying elements from which we derive coordinates in geography, dates in history, ranking in family lineage, and hence track all vertical and horizontal stressors (key forming factors) in a person's life. Only through understanding numbers will we become at peace with ourselves, for simply through this understanding we will recognize that we are not alone and, more importantly, cure ourselves of rabies.

Rabies is a virus transmitted to humans via bites, sometimes from humans. Once infected, humans manifest neurologic symptoms, such as alternating periods of aggression, anxiety, normal behavior, and depression. Typically, rabid humans are shown to drool because the salivary glands are infected and the jaws become paralyzed, which makes them appear to foam at the mouth. Eventually, the violence subsides and the human dies after a period of disorientation. Could a more indolent form of this virus be more widespread than is known, infecting societies at large and has a prolonged cycle with less apparent salivary symptoms?

Browsing through statistics, we should start seeing how many live their lives: never to marry, marry but never have children, marry and get divorced (with or without children), healthy, disabled, are born as orphans, wish to be orphans, etc. And here we are using binary outcomes. You can either marry or not; there is no in-between state. Alternatively, we also should recognize how much one can earn money, wealth in general, friends, enemies, intimate relationships, devour quantities of food, sleep endless hours, and others. Here, however, the outcome is a continuous number—with decimal points, if you want. However, in the midst of all this, we should realize the factors that determine how happy and contented we are. Subsequently, we should be humble when we consider the probability to achieve the maximum in all the continuous predictors and seek/maintain positive one of all the binaries. Overlapping all the curves onto you is really an infinitesimally small probability. A probability is that all the unrealistic rabies infected act as if they are promised to achieve. Hence, they live at a hurried pace, scoring themselves based on an external scale and opening themselves to judgment, seeking external validation, and are ultimately set to fail because they do not recognize that they are a success as they are at each time point. Alternatively, the believers and self-confident call this low probability "hope" and work for it open only to his judgment.

We stand to attest our belonging to the class of healers—unique and never was or to recur—and simultaneously to attest to the outcome of an infinitesimally small probability of a binary outcome that is continuously evolving and cured of rabies (fluctuations of anxiety, anger, depression, paralyzed muscles, and foaming teeth) by the power of understanding numbers, guided by the Primary, and contented with ourselves as we are.

Blessed is he who knows his worth and limits, and works in accordance. Determine yours, and recognize that our blessings are innumerable.

Outcome-based Healing Approach: From Prophecy to Artificial Intelligence

Hussain Isma'eel and Imad Elhajj

The core reason individuals will seek your healing abilities is their belief that with you, they can heal successfully. This relationship is centered on them trusting you to help them and guide them to the favorable outcome they desire. *It is an outcome-based relationship.* Naturally, in this loop, you as a healer are both affecting and affected. In each transaction, you are modulating your approach (learning) to deliver healing, and with that, the relationship is also evolving either to be positively reinforced (good outcome) or otherwise (bad outcome). It is a feedback loop.

It is important to highlight that in this process, we as healers are providing our synthesis (recommendations) *as experts acting as coaches for decision making mainly_and in very limited occasions as decision takers.* The differentiation between the two roles is important because this is the difference between those who want to abuse their expertise to reverse the situation and become mostly or always decision takers. This is what we are not. The reason we are not this is because we genuinely understand: *The outcome desired, i.e., healing, does not have the same face for all of us.* For some individuals, risk avoiding and living whatever remains of their days in a happy manner and permitting the natural course of the disease is healing. For others, risk taking in hopes of altering the natural course of the disease is their understanding of healing. We should respect that healing has different meanings, and it is fundamentally based on each individual's belief system.

Understanding this, we are not dictators, and our patients are not expected to be compliant. Compliance is a passive process used to describe rubber bands. Our patients are humans with beliefs, predilections, will, and decision making capabilities. Hence, we should be, mostly, coaches to promote adherence to behaviors that to our best knowledge, i.e., "expertise," will lead to healing according to our patients' satisfaction. The definition of healing is something individuals need to answer for themselves.

To illustrate:

Situation dictates the best approach to follow

Situation	Our approach	Outcome
Chronic diseases followed up in the clinic requiring 1. Smoking cessation 2. Adherence to chronic medications (statins, anticoagulants) 3. Lifestyle changes including exercising 4. Dietary changes	Coach Decision taker	Favorable Unfavorable

Time critical

1. A dissection occurred during a coronary angioplasty	Coach	Might lead to patient death
2. An artery is bleeding as a complication of an operation and the patient is on the operating table	Decision taker	Life saving

Conflict between autonomy and beneficence

1. A gentleman with delirium and refusing treatment for sepsis	Coach	Unethical and can lead to patient death
	Decision taker	Ethical and can save the patient

Alternatively, one of the toughest situations you as a healer might be involved in is to guide the patient and the family to understand the concept of futility of an intervention. Medical futility refers to interventions that are unlikely to produce any significant benefit for the patient. Two kinds of medical futility are often distinguished.

- *Quantitative futility, where the likelihood (hence the quantitative component in it) that an intervention will benefit the patient is extremely poor, and*
- *Qualitative futility, where the quality of benefit (supposing the patient survives the intervention with no complications) an intervention will produce is extremely poor.*

Both quantitative and qualitative futility refer to the prospect of benefiting the patient (the outcome). A treatment that mostly improves

the patient's numbers (urine output or blood pressure, for example)
and does not necessarily lead to any benefit that the patient can
appreciate is futile. Again, since our interventions (ranging from
counseling to open heart surgery) are outcome driven, we must have
a clear mind regarding where/what this intervention can lead to.
Without knowing the outcome and clearly stating that to the patient
and the family, how can you expect them to make a well-informed
decision? Similarly, without us knowing the patient, the family, and
their culture, how can we understand their decision to carry on with
certain interventions that we (based on our knowledge and culture)
might deem futile or, conversely, refuse interventions that in our
opinion lead to favorable outcomes? This is the challenge that we
prepare to deal with: making sure that we *intervene in an outcome-*
and evidence-based manner and that our outcome is healing the
patient, not eliminating the disease. Eliminating the disease may or
may not accompany healing.

From a historical perspective and to further reinforce the significance
of our role, we ask you to reflect on the word "prophecy" and how
close it is to the word "prognosis." While the latter is the word we use
in medical jargon to refer to prediction of the course of the patient's
interaction with illness such as death or survival course, the former is
used in religious and literary jargon to refer to prediction of outcomes.
Hence, it is important that we recognize that, given our abilities that
can to a certain degree of accuracy predict outcomes, our patients
perceive that we possess the power to foresee their future. Hence, we
are capable of helping them minimize uncertainty in the future in
regards to their health. We are providing them with recommendations
that help appease the anxiety of the unknown through making it
known to a certain degree of accuracy. Based on the prognosis we
provide them, they go back and manage their lives. What we provide
impacts our patients at many levels.

Mr. ML was a 60-year-old gentleman on the ward for workup for
a lung mass. He was a very well-read gentleman who worked as a
senior banker. While being worked up, the medical student heard
a heart murmur that was associated with shortness of breath with
exercise. An echocardiography revealed severe aortic stenosis. In
the meantime, the result of the lung mass workup came back, which

indicated the patient has advanced nonoperable lung cancer. Mr. ML was not yet aware of the lung cancer and was persistently asking questions about the valve and how it can be managed, such as the type of surgery he needed, the type of valve (mechanical or biological) he should get, and the advantages of each choice. Once he was informed about the existence of lung cancer, there was a complete shift in the questions, and they all were reduced to one: "Which will kill me first?" As a banker, and like all intelligent humans, he wanted to know the time course of his illness so he can prioritize. "Proper management in life includes proper time management and prioritization," he said. He lived according to a motto he was taught earlier: Blessed is he who knows where he is, where he was and where he is heading.

Accordingly, he wanted to know so he can write his will and perform many things that he has been postponing. "A human changes when he knows for real that his death is imminent," he said, "And I am glad that at least I have some time to do the things I would like to do."

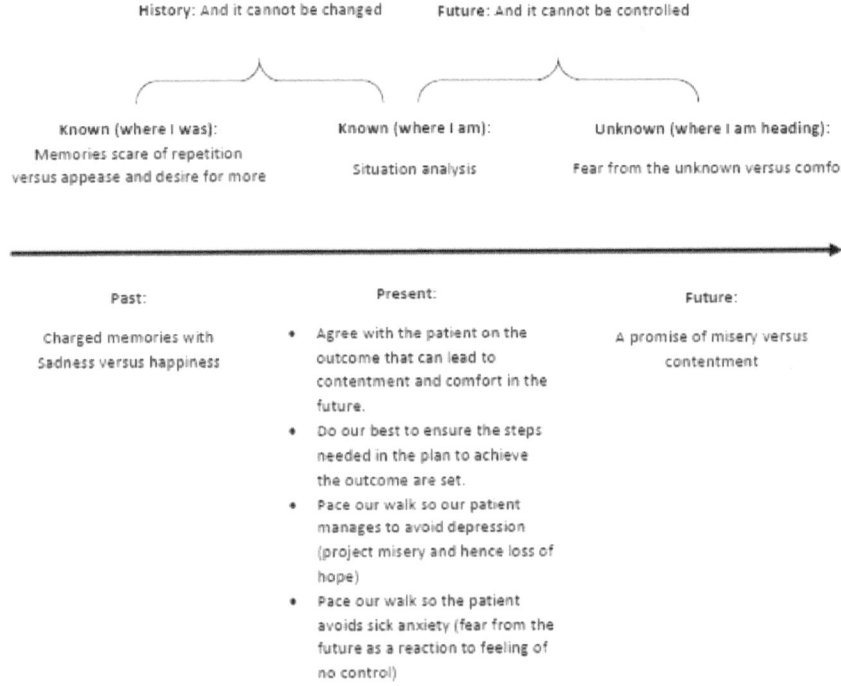

History: And it cannot be changed   Future: And it cannot be controlled

Known (where I was):
Memories scare of repetition versus appease and desire for more

Known (where I am):
Situation analysis

Unknown (where I am heading):
Fear from the unknown versus comfort

Past:
Charged memories with Sadness versus happiness

Present:
- Agree with the patient on the outcome that can lead to contentment and comfort in the future.
- Do our best to ensure the steps needed in the plan to achieve the outcome are set.
- Pace our walk so our patient manages to avoid depression (project misery and hence loss of hope)
- Pace our walk so the patient avoids sick anxiety (fear from the future as a reaction to feeling of no control)

Future:
A promise of misery versus contentment

In the figure above, we illustrate the concepts discussed earlier. We simply accompany our patients in a journey, providing them a promise that we are guides to make the best choices now to reach the outcome in the unknown (the future). We help our patients decrease their sadness from their current situation, not feel sad about their past, and provide some guidance on how to minimize their pain and agony so they are not miserable in the future. Should the patient feel melancholic, look backwards, and feel low, then project forward and become gloomy, then this patient is heading for depression—if he is not already depressed. Similarly, if the patient currently feels scared of the illness, looks backwards, and feels sad about what he missed in the past, and if he also feels scared, fearful, and weary, and becomes indecisive when looking forward, then this patient is now caught by a paralyzing anxiety. We should be the patient's guide to enable decision making and ameliorate the patient's anxiety. We are the patient's guide to the desired outcome by providing the patient a sense of orientation as to the current situation, where this might have possibly started from, and what to do for a better future. This is a glimpse of the outcome-based understanding of our role.

Traditionally, we in the medical sciences have relied on certain statistical methods to predict outcomes. Briefly, all these methods work on correlating certain features of patients and their illness with the outcome that we are interested in. The regression method is probably among the most commonly used, and the Kaplan–Meier survival curves are the most famous in medical literature. Recently, however, more powerful mathematical modeling and increased computational power has enabled the creation of newer and in some cases more accurate tools to predict outcome. The vision is for these tools to be part of the branch of science referred to as artificial intelligence (AI). This branch of science involves creating intelligent machines or machines that can sense the exterior, make sense of it, and then make decisions that maximize chances of success to achieve the desired outcome. In a way, this science is trying to create machines that replicate what we as healers do. Hence, this is what is envisioned as "the future doctor." Those of you who watch science fiction are the most capable of relating to this when they remember famous robots. Of course, we are still far from this, but remember that Jules Verne wrote about the journey to the moon hundreds of years before that was done, which was less than 70 years ago. We are now witnessing journeys to Mars. AI currently has tools in clinical practice (some already exist as smartphone applications). The fundamental added value from these tools is their increased accuracy in predicting the outcome after being "taught" the historical data. We must be open and aware of the existence of these tools and that there are more of them to come. Thus, we should be able to understand these tools to properly utilize them.

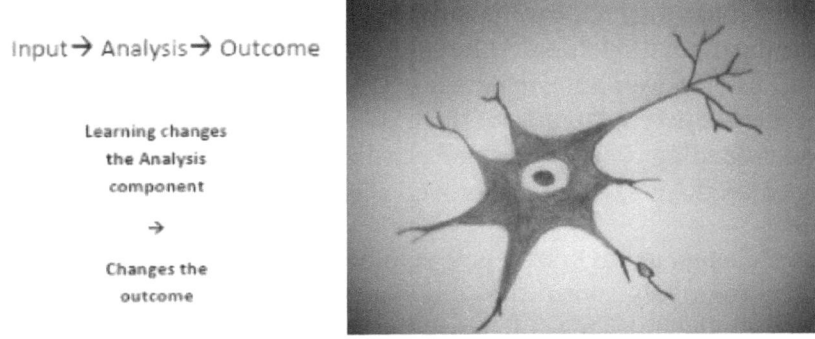

Input → Analysis → Outcome

Learning changes
the Analysis
component

→

Changes the
outcome

Figure by MA. Al Masri

Several such techniques have evolved in the field of artificial intelligence and pattern recognition. Some of the most currently popular methods are support vector machines (SVM) and artificial neural network (ANN). Among the various mathematical modeling methods, we want to introduce the ANN model. As its name implies, ANN was inspired by the way our neurons interact to learn and recognize patterns. From our neuroscience course, we remember that the end result of a circuit of neurons is not the same each time a stimulus arrives. For example, in neural circuits, there is the phenomenon of potentiating where repetitive stimuli predispose the postsynaptic neuron to fire at lower thresholds. In other words, the postsynaptic neuron "learned" to fire at a lower threshold. Hence, the interaction between a stimulus and an outcome may have been linear in the beginning, but later it became different, requiring a lower intensity to activate the postsynaptic neuron and generate the outcome. Similarly, ANN-based models evolve (learn) the more information is provided (the more training) to improve the accuracy of a predicted outcome. Therefore, relationships that were linear in the beginning may end up being not linear with more data. However, a balance has to be drawn between training and overtraining, as overtraining might result in the model fitting the training data too well and thus lose its ability to extrapolate.

ANN has two main advantages over regression: Nonlinearity (or linearity) is learned from the data, and the relationship between the input and outcome evolves as more data are used to train, and hidden ones may appear that may not be linear or may have complex nonlinear relationships. Other modeling methods exist, and each one has its power and advantages. We are not expected to learn how these were derived or master them. We are expected to have a general understanding and also properly utilize the tools that are generated based on them to ensure improved accuracy in predicting outcomes.

We are expected to know enough to be able to collaborate efficiently and effectively with the engineers, computer scientists, and mathematicians. This collaboration, which is a must in this day and age, would result in better outcome prediction. We cannot keep using the tools of the past only to predict the future when our present has changed. Just as our lives have evolved with increased risk factors, our tools must evolve in order to model more complex relationships between symptoms, diseases, and outcomes. We would not be doing our patients any favor if we don't evolve our tools. Frankly, it would be borderline unethical if we don't take the time (which is your most precious resource) to exploit advances in AI, modeling, and technology in general for the betterment of outcome prediction and other aspects of healthcare.

Case Example

The concept of outcome-based interventions is now widely recognized in the field. It is rooted in what is commonly known as evidence-based medical practice. To elaborate, consider the following:

Mr. CS is a 55-year-old gentleman with hypertension that is well controlled and is a 30-pack-year smoker, dyslipidemic on treatment with a statin, and his current total cholesterol is 230 mg/dl with LDL 120 mg/dl. He is presenting to your clinic for a routine checkup. His history is completely negative for any chest discomfort, and his physical exam is benign with a systolic blood pressure of 138/88 mmHg. He tells you he has read that he is at high risk for coronary artery disease and would like to undergo a test that helps determine if he has coronary artery disease. You recommend

    a. Stress echocardiography
    b. Coronary CT angiography
    c. Stress nuclear
    d. Nothing

Based on the above case, what the patient is requesting appears reasonable. To determine what to do, we need to ask ourselves the following:

1. In a population of patients similar to this, how many will have a positive stress test and how many will not?
2. Among those who have a positive stress test, how many will end up with significant coronary artery disease?
3. Should we take this segment with asymptomatic individuals and have them undergo stress testing to uncover silent coronary artery disease and then have them undergo angioplasty, what is their outcome relative to those who are treated medically only? (Outcome is either death from cardiovascular diseases or a composite outcome of death or myocardial infarction.)

Answering Q1 will inform you how much this intervention leads to incurred cost to identify a relatively small segment.

Answering Q2 will inform you how much the false positive rate of the chosen stress test will lead to unwarranted cardiac catheterizations.

Answering Q3 will inform you that medical therapy to control the traditional modifiable risk factors (hypertension, dyslipidemia, smoking, lack of exercise, diabetes, etc.) in this patient leads to a similar outcome than the entire cascade of events in the track that is followed.

This is the background of the recommendation of the cardiology societies against performing stress nuclear, coronary CT angiography, or stress echocardiography in asymptomatic individuals. *The results of these interventions do not alter the final outcome.* Thus, the answer is none of the above; just treat the modifiable risk factors. Anything done otherwise is a loss of money, time, and effort and causes unwarranted concerns to the patient. Only by giving the patients enough time to explain the above steps and the risks of every procedure will the patients agree to the recommendation. We are aware that some physicians find this concept difficult to adhere to, so we should not be surprised if patients show some skepticism too.

A person in all places: the past, the present and the future at once

When I was young, I used to play soccer. In that game, I always wanted to be the midfield player. That was out of an understanding of my abilities, for I was 80% defender and attacker, and therefore neither 100% striker nor could I tolerate being 100% defender. However, at crucial moments, I had it in me to return to the defensive line and just slide in front of the opponent, or alternatively support the offensive and even shoot at the goal when the opportunity is there. Hence, my abilities were in line with this role, for I was one of those who would run all the game, be very happy with receiving from the defenders to pass to our attackers, and be ready to be where needed. I knew my place and it was known to others too!

Here, take a moment and reflect, and you will see that you are like me, but in different games. In some, we are the midfield players. In others, we are the defenders or the attackers—and sometimes just watching from the sidelines—also as in life. Since I used to play this game every Wednesday and Thursday, I was refining and learning about our opponents (who were usually from a competing school) and working with my team (who were usually from my school). Thus, I was improving, for I was learning from the past's mistakes, applying in the present—to become the past in a moment—and shaping the future all at once. Isn't this what you do when you react to a behavior from someone you love, someone you hate, or someone just new and unknown? You and I would be in all moments at once.

This is true in all things: in soccer, medicine, cooking, drinking and eating habits, driving cars, and in everything else, particularly with humans. I was taught, "Blessed are those who know where they are, where they were, and where they are heading."

I admit, however, that sometimes this threefold existence was imbalanced, for I would be at school in class—the present—daydreaming of what I wanted to be—the future—forgetting that every time I would do this, I would not understand the lecture—and it has just become the past! Or I would be in a party, with loud noises, and get carried away in the moment—the present—forgetting what I had learned—the past—and ending up with a car accident, hence altering my future! But worse (something I have now learned to do on my own in the right time), I would indulge in analyzing the past, forgetting the present and thus severely affecting the future. Balancing this threefold existence is what keeps me alert and present. Thus, I simply I exist.

Healing: INDEX

Hussain Isma'eel and Wissam Alajaji

Objectives

After reading this chapter, a medical student should acquire the following:

1. *Develop communication skills pertinent to the medical encounter*
2. *Learn how to get to know the patient rather than the disease and be a good listener*
3. *Be introduced to the concept of individualizing medical care as far as testing and treatment options depending on patient background variability*
4. *Introduced to evidence-based thinking in the decision making of hospital admission*
5. *Develop a strategy to go through the process of narrowing down a differential diagnosis*

To help the student achieve a successful medical encounter, we developed the INDEX acronym (see page 78). The INDEX acronym should help remind the medical student about key points pertinent to history, the patient interview, differential diagnosis, and patient triage. During the course of this chapter, we detail the INDEX acronym, and we hope the reader will find this concept helpful.

Index

Now that you are open to receive your role, let's prove that we can perform it. Like any new encounter, you will need all your senses to be ready to receive. In the beginning, we need you to listen to, inquire about, and feel your patient's pain and concerns. In doing so, you are now in the "I" of the INDEX, embracing your patient's "I" and seeing him through yours (reflecting). The main objective is to be *intensely in touch with your patient* and therefore quantitatively and qualitatively assess the intensity of his/her illness and feelings. *The goal is to develop jointly a plan to heal.*

In the scheme below, you will start with listening and inquiring about the patient's symptoms' qualitative and quantitative aspects. To simplify things, in brief, you are asking:

Who is the patient?

What is the patient's complaint?

When did this complaint first appear and its temporal characteristics?

Where is the area of concern, and what does the physical exam show?

The HOW stands for: the head (alertness and level of consciousness) and hemodynamics (blood pressure, heart rate, respiratory rate), the O2 saturation, and the water, i.e., hydration status (edematous versus hypovolemic).

- **Who: demographics and past medical Hx**
- **What: subjective symptoms**
- **When: temporal aspects**
- **Where: physical exam**
- **HOW: head and hemodynamics, O2, water (hydration)**

However, if we restrict our inquiries to that, then we have cut the communication bridge. Do not sever this bridge, but instead try to get to know the value system of your patients and acknowledge it. Once they feel respected, they will reciprocate respect and acknowledgment. This is part of what will increase your value in their eyes (over and above your clinical skills), and the more you do of that, the more you will be seen as distinguished. This is the beginning of parting away from the "regular" medical doctor path. Do we care if our patient is single and lives alone or not, or is a believer in God or not? Very gently, try to do the following:

1. Ask what the patient does for a living or what his/her hobbies are. The profession and hobby will help you identify the jargon the patient can best relate to. For example:
    a. With bankers – "Let's try to *maximize your return* from your visit with me"; "If you *invest* some effort in the . . . you will *de-risk* your situation"; and so on so forth.
    b. With housewives – "Write your prescription yourself. It's your *recipe* in your own cookbook for a healthier life."
    c. With a basketball fan - Use words like "three points," "slam dunk," etc.
2. Try to understand in the most subtle way whether or not you are dealing with a believer in God or not. This will help you understand how much this individual sees an afterlife or not. With people who believe and see an afterlife, speak to them using terms such as peace, relief, warmth, and good deeds. With those who believe in karma, say things like "Whatever you do will come back to you." The latter statement applies to both believers of God and karma.
3. Try to comprehend and envision that the person in front of you is coming with a "bent back" (figuratively speaking, kyphotic or even scoliotic) from the burden of disease. This is extremely important for the purpose of motivating the patient to adhere to therapy, and more so when the diseases are chronic (hypertension, diabetes, etc.) and entail life changes. Your duty is to help him uplift himself. Let him first express this feeling (this is when they are open to receive) and directly use words such as, "You are strong and this will not break your back nor should you look down." You can even ask them

to write down on a piece of paper, "I am strong, and I can overcome this."

We will not expand further on communication here as there will be a chapter for that. However, the practice follows the following principle:

"Prophets, men of the word, were ordered to speak people's language/words to modernize them and motivate them forward."

Try to reflect on this statement, for *you are a carrier of a message of healing*, and therefore you are a mini-prophet in our domain. *Determine your domain, so you dominate it.*

Once the sensual (listening, observing, and feeling) part of the proactive process of "I" has been exhausted, it is time for more proactivity, i.e., to probe and react. In fact, this process has been ongoing since the patient decided to come to you, and you decided to show up. You shall see that later.

Probing allows us to acquire more pertinent information about the patient's illness. This is done usually through imaging and lab tests.

Here, you should answer the following questions in this order:

1. Arrange the differential diagnosis list from the most probable to the least probable as per your analysis. This is neither easy not difficult. Usually, we seem to put high on the list what we objectively think is high, and then we include the low item on the list what we know is low, but we are scared to exclude anything because the outcomes of missing this might be detrimental. This will be further elaborated in (2).
2. *What* is the best tool to confirm/negate the possibility of a disease? Central to this is to know the negative and positive likelihood ratios of the tests you order. The latter is because these numbers will help you quantify to the patient the probability of having or not having the disease. This will serve as a key for justifying to the patient and third-party payers *why* a certain test is ordered, and for communicating the message

in the Expectations section later. Furthermore, the PLR and NLR are universal in the sense that these numbers should not change with the prevalence of the disease across different genders or ethnicities. Hence, you can memorize them once and be done with them. These numbers will change with the improvement in the technology you are utilizing, so make sure to know *what tool is available at* your center.

Which test? Can he/she do it? When to do it?

What tool is available at your center is of prime importance to know because individuals have different needs. For example, a claustrophobic patient cannot undergo an MRI, which takes place in a closed machine, and an obese individual might not fit in the CT or MRI. Similarly, a person with severe knee osteoarthritis or a limp cannot undergo a treadmill exercise test. A person with elevated creatinine or iodine allergy should not receive intravenous contrast material. Knowing what tool you have and *who operates it* and *their level of experience* will help you decide whether *the patient should undergo this test* and *if the patient can undergo this test* using this tool.

The sequence of tests to be ordered (*when to do the test and which batch of tests to order first*) should follow the following balanced position:

Order the test with the lowest NLR for the least probable disease on your differential (the one at the bottom of the list), and order the test with the highest PLR for the disease you listed as the top of your suspects. If you do so, then you will avoid missing the least common (which is sometimes fatal, like a myocardial infarction in a young gentleman) and also accelerate confirming that the top suspect is the cause of illness, respectively.

iNdex

Navigation

```
┌──────────────────────────────────────────────────────────┐
│ Where: outpatient, inpatient (ward vs. critical care) – safe setting │
│ Who: transferring team – safe transfer                     │
│ When: proper timing (indicators of safe timing)            │
│ HOW: safe means (defibrillator, etc.)                      │
└──────────────────────────────────────────────────────────┘
```

The question of where to and how are we are transferring the patient for continuity of care is guided by the principle "patient safety is prime." Secondary to this principle is the cost savings concern, which is important but not prime. Therefore, a balanced position would be one that addresses both in accordance to their weight, i.e., a value-weighted decision. To implement this, we need to start with the following questions:

Questions set A

1. What is the severity/intensity of the patient's condition?
2. From 1, what is the near-term prognosis?
3. What is the outcome measured by the prognosis?
4. What are the accuracy/limitations of this tool?

The questions above help frame our thought flow to determine the best choice. Ideally, to answer these questions, we should look for a tool that does that. We elaborate this situation by using the case of pneumonia. Several tools for scoring pneumonia risk exist. CURB 65 is probably among the simplest and earliest tools developed by W. Lim et al, Thorax. 2003 May; 58(5): 377–382. The acronym stands for confusion by AMT (abbreviated mental test score of $<= 8$), urea greater than 19 mg/dl, respiratory rate $>= 30$/min, SBP< 90 mmHg or DBP<60 mmHg, age $>= 65$. For every item, one point is given, and then the points are summed up and a corresponding risk for death at 30 days is given with a suggested disposition direction (Table 1).

Table 1 CURB 65 SCORE to predict risk of death at 30 days from pneumonia and disposition

Score	Risk of death at 30 days	Disposition
0–1	0.7% to 3.2%	Outpatient
2–3	13% to 17%	Short stay at hospital or close observation at home
4–5	41.5% to 57%	Hospitalization, possibly ICU

Table 1 shows that the measured outcome is death. The first thing one should think of is "What about other outcomes, such as respiratory failure leading to brain anoxia?" After all, this is a disastrous outcome that can impact negatively not only the patient, but also the family and the treating physician and the hospital in terms of medico-legal consequences. Furthermore, the outcome measured is at 30 days, while we are interested in a shorter term outcome to guide a *now* decision to answer where the patient should be sent. Moreover, the accuracy of the CURB 65 has been shown to be limited with an area under the receiving operator curve (AU-ROC) of 0.63. According to statistics, the latter number corresponds to poor accuracy. Hence, what we have is a tool that is far from optimal. Other more refined tools have been introduced, and they include more variables and outcomes, and are more accurate in answering short-term questions.

However, the aim of this section is to provide guidance and a general framework that is applicable to the majority of diseases. *This is to be followed in conjunction with adherence to the appropriate medical guidelines and not to replace or forget them.* We think the following scheme is helpful, and it follows the *iAMOSMS acronym, which stands for: illness, age, mental status (abbreviated mental* *test score of <= 8), organ-specific indicators, systemic indicators, morbidities/medications, and system of support (Table 2).* These components were chosen out of careful observations and are guided by the following principles:

1. The most important predictor of death remains to be age.
2. An altered mental status indicates increased patient risk for aspiration/bedsores, advanced illness, and increased difficulty in caring for the patient at home.
3. The illness in most situations originates from an organ, and therapy always targets this organ. Therefore, organ-specific indicators showing a heavily damaged organ are compelling reasons to warrant more attention and care (e.g., multilobar pneumonia, lung crackles reaching upper 1/3 of lung in CHF, super elevated liver enzymes in hepatitis).
4. Once an organ is affected, a systemic reaction ensues. More care is warranted if extreme reactions are observed, such as an elevated Cr, very high fever, hypotension or severe hypertension, tachypnea or hypopnea, >80% age-predicted maximum heart rate or bradycardia, hypoxia on room air or very high white blood cell count, and hypo or hyperkalemia. Extreme reactions are better addressed in the hospital.
5. Morbidities count in terms of quality and quantity. The more immune modulating and systemic is the comorbidity; a worse disease status indicates that more care should be given. On the other hand, more numerous comorbidities indicates that the therapy is more challenging in terms of drug-drug interactions, adherence, drug fever, and increased risk of errors.
6. Support system refers to who receives the patient. If a patient with a borderline moderate severity illness that could deteriorate is going to be sent home where he/she is alone, then this is inappropriate. Similarly, assigning an ill patient who can deteriorate to a regular floor and leaving him unsupervised is also inappropriate. Conversely, ICU beds are reserved for those in need, and hospitalizations are costly. *Note that patient safety is prime.* Therefore, a plan that optimizes patient's needs is the best option. Be caring, inquisitive, and resourceful to offer solutions. A home nurse

may be covered by insurance or be a more cost-efficient option to avoid hospitalization for an insured or self-paying person who lives alone, respectively. An in-hospital accompanying nurse may also be useful to avoid sending the patient to the ICU or compromising his care.

How and when to transfer

The navigation direction has been determined. What remains to be decided now is how and when. This bears repeating: *patient safety is prime; cost savings is secondary; and in haste is error.*

The behaviors commensurate with the above start with answering the question:

What are the red flags in the iAMOSMS scheme that swayed us to admit this patient?

After identifying the red flags, the following needs to be done:

1. Proper communication with the receiving party ensures that the patient is well received and the setting is appropriate. *Use the iIAMOSMS scheme to deliver the message in the order of: Mr. or Ms. is a case of ...i....and is A...y.o.....M....O....S....M/M......S......*

    Highlight the red flags that pushed you to decide to admit the patient. The recipient will then see the case through your eyes and therefore have a concordant evaluation of the gravity of the situation.

2. In the absence of a label of high acuity by the emergency department team, recognizing what led us to decide to admit from the IAMOSMS scheme (the red flags) will determine the outcomes we are working hard to avoid. Naturally, *these red flags also need to be avoided in the journey. These are mostly related to the mental and systemic components of the iAMOSMS scheme, in particular, heart rate, blood pressure, and respiratory rate and O2 saturation. Precautions to*

prevent and deal with them should they occur need to be present with the transferring team.

For example:

Case of COPD exacerbation

Consider that you are seeing a 50-year-old gentleman known to have moderate COPD and has been treated and stabilized in the ED. However, he remains tachypneic and hypoxic on room air, but is in an acceptable situation on 3l O2 with O2 90% saturation.

This individual needs to be accompanied with an intubation set and oxygen in addition to the crash kit and pulse oxymeter.

In cases labeled as high acuity by the emergency department team, the system in place should be the one with the highest safety. Adhere to this system; this is safer for everybody, including you.

3. Timing of transfer is also determined by the iAMOSMS scheme. First, identify the red flags. Then, ask yourself:

    a. How imminent is each catastrophe (red flag)?
    b. How can we best prevent this event?
    c. Should this event occur, where is the best place for this to be attended to?

Answering these three questions will tell you if this is the right time to transfer the patient or not.

For example:

Case of GI bleeding

Consider that you are seeing a 65-year-old gentleman with excessive GI bleeding who is vomiting blood and is hypotensive (SBP 70 mm Hg) and tachycardic (HR 130 bpm).

As per the IAMOSMS, the red flag here is pending arrest secondary to blood loss.

Answer to Q1: Very imminent

Answer to Q2: The ABCs of urgent care first and foremost, i.e., volume expansion and blood transfusions

Answer to Q3: In the ED first for stabilizing before transferring to the endoscopy suite

inDex

The D component of the INDEX is probably the most overarching part in the INDEX scheme. This is because we are always developing our understanding of the patient's condition, and development is part of all the other components. With each piece of information, we are either modulating our approach, negating a possibility on our differential, further validating an etiology, or completely changing our direction. We need to underscore that the anchoring component of this arch is patient consent. Without this, we deny that the patient is a deciding entity, and this clearly deviates from the path of healers.

1. **Therapeutic – focused on the #1 priority/1' disease**
2. **Supportive/palliative (ABCs and PAIN and LAXATIVES)**
3. **Preventive (prophylactic measures)**
4. **Consent**

As soon as the history taking and physical exam sections are completed, a therapeutic plan is developed. This plan should respect a certain order highlighted in the box above. The order is to be respected in terms of flow only. The consent component is not the least important at all; on the contrary, it is the part that wraps up everything. Consent indicates that the patient was informed and is in agreement.

The best case to illustrate this is the case of a patient presenting with chest pain.

Mr. CP is presenting with chest pain to the ED. He is a 45-year-old gentleman who is alert and can provide a reliable history. He describes his chest pain as sharp and retro-sternal, and that it lasted for five minutes and woke him up from sleep. This is the first time he has experienced such a pain. The pain was relieved spontaneously and was not associated with palpitations, sweating, shortness of breath, or loss of consciousness. His vital signs and physical exam do not reveal any abnormality. He is a smoker, but not a known diabetic or hypertensive, nor does he have a history of vascular diseases. He is not on any chronic medications except for aspirin, which he takes by himself for cardiac protection as he has a family history of sudden death; his father passed away at the age of 43 from a cardiac arrest. He was brought in by his wife, who is now taking care of the insurance paperwork, and they left their three kids at home alone. The eldest child is 12 years old.

Note that the case presentation followed the iAMSOMS scheme. Revisit it to confirm this to yourself and practice writing this.

T

Following the steps above, we should then focus on the number one priority, i.e., the cause of the patient's chief complaint. We intentionally did not want to complicate this case by introducing other findings or morbidities. However, once these are observed, we need to be able to prioritize. How we prioritize can also be derived from the iAMOSMS scheme. *In brief, any red flag that has been highlighted in the iAMSOMS scheme or is the factor in the admission of the patient should be attended to.* To avoid redundancy, we will not repeat this here; refer to the section above on navigation. Here, we are primarily concerned about myocardial infarction or death. Therefore, our plan needs to address this.

S

The first batch of results is out. The minute a test turns out negative, we are prompted to put this possible etiology linked to this test low on the differential. How low depends on the NLR of the test: the lower the etiology, the more confident we are in ruling out disease. Conversely, should the results of a test turn out to be positive, then the etiology is shifted upward in the differential. Depending on the PLR of the test used, if this test is positive, then we either pursue this etiology with high confidence and initiate treatment (if the posttest probability is high) or request another test with a higher PLR, which is usually the reference standard test (if the posttest probability is high but not enough to initiate treatment).

1. Among the first batch of tests physicians order are an ECG and a troponin test.
2. If the ECG is normal, then this is not a ST elevation myocardial infarction, but this does not mean this is neither non-ST elevation MI nor unstable angina. This is where the ECG serves as the reference test with the lowest NLR and highest PLR for STEMI. Of importance to know that this case is so because of the nomenclature, that is, the definition is based on the ECG. However, the ECG's NLR and PLR for

NSTEMI or unstable angina is suboptimal, which is why we cannot rely on one single ECG to consider or rule out the latter conditions.

3. If the troponin is normal, then we know for now that this is less likely to be an NSTEMI. However, it could still be an NSTEMI or unstable angina.

4. Once the second set of troponin is out after six hours, we are more confident that this is not NSTEMI, and the only explanation that remains is unstable angina.

5. Conversely, should the troponin turn out to be positive, then the posttroponin result probability of NSTEMI is high. Therefore, the approach is modulated, and the patient is admitted to the cardiac unit. *Note that we say high probability without certainty because there are numerous causes for falsely elevated troponin.*

6. However, should the second set of troponin turn out to be negative, then we are faced with the important question: What if this is unstable angina? We are then placed in a situation that requires working our way through a rule-out coronary artery disease event track that is very similar to the process above but using another test (stress testing or CT coronary angiography are usually utilized for low-intermediate pretest probability of coronary event).

indEx

Re-emphasizing the outcome-based approach in medical practice, setting expectations is important for both the patient and us as healers. Based on our previous knowledge of the outcome of patients with similar conditions to that of the patient we are working with, we can predict the trend our patient will follow depending on different routes and interventions we agree with the patient to follow/undertake. This is central to all our practice, from recognizing what is the best intervention to obtaining consent. Without this, we are operating in darkness and have little to offer our patients.

Let us take Mr. CP's case that we discussed in the previous section one step further as an example. After two sets of troponin turned out negative, with the absence of ECG changes, and without recurrence of chest pain, the possibility of Mr. CP dying or having a myocardial infarction within the coming two to four weeks becomes quite low. Actually, this is what the TIMI risk scoring system permits us to predict and relay to the patient. Based on this expectation, we and the patient need to agree on the next step. Given that the probability of a coronary event is now low and following the logic we discussed earlier in the "Power of the Tool" section, what we should aim for is to rule out a coronary event, i.e., to go with a test that has the lowest possible NLR. What we are doing here is simply taking someone who to start with had a low likelihood of disease to nearly zero likelihood of coronary disease. This is the logic followed in the current rule-out protocol in emergency departments and chest pain units.

On the other hand, we should be very realistic from the beginning and recognize that since we are starting from a low likelihood of disease, even if the result of the test we chose to rule out turns out to be positive for obstructive coronary disease, the posttest likelihood for disease will remain relatively low. In other words, we will have a high rate of false positives. This again follows the Bayesian nomogram discussed earlier.

With that explained, it is only normal then that these rule-out protocols are going to lead to a very high number of true negatives and false positives. This raises the question of proper utilization of these tests and the issue of cost effectiveness. Pending a more cost-conscious and better screening methods to determine within the low pretest probability cases who should we send to further testing, this is the best we have to offer our patients. Denying our patients this protocol is synonymous to saying that the 5% of patients who will have a myocardial infarction or die within 30 days from discharge from the emergency department with negative serial ECGs and troponins are not worth the cost.

indeX

One of the paths that Mr. CP can follow is to undergo the rule-out test (for example, a stress nuclear study), and the result turns out to be positive for obstructive coronary artery disease. At this moment, a whole new set of extra factors comes into the equation. These factors can be approached using the DONE acronym highlighted below.

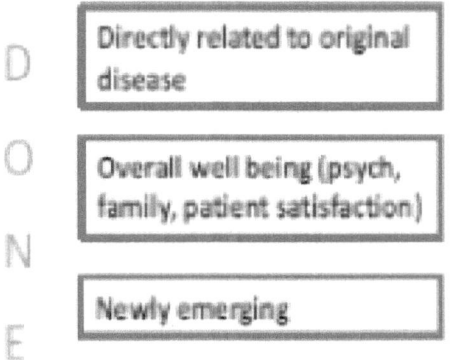

D   Directly related to original disease

O   Overall well being (psych, family, patient satisfaction)

N

E   Newly emerging

Certain examples include the following:

D – Directly related to his disease: Mr. CP now needs to be admitted for a cardiac catheterization. However, he has a remote history of iodine allergy. Therefore, we need to discuss the benefits and risks of the procedure on the patient. This also requires Mr. CP to take time off from work, which might coincide with some of his deadlines. However, Mr. CP has a set of questions he wants to ask: What is the impact of this on my insurance premiums? Will I have to change my job, which entails a significant amount of stress and physical labor? If I do, then what is going to happen to my income, and how will that affect my family's overall (O) well-being? Should I need to insert a scaffold to open a clogged artery, does this mean antiplatelets for life?

In brief, the result of one test has put Mr. CP on a life-changing course. We as healers should understand the gravity of this change and be ready and well equipped to guide our patient and his family in this transitional period. Attending to these concerns and empathizing with the patient is what will ensure the patient's satisfaction from his interaction with you as a healer and the institution at large.

To further highlight the importance of the above, we must remind ourselves that while the truth is that the majority of our patients will cope with this transition, it is also true that some will not and will develop either anxiety or depression (newly emerging factors). Early recognition of the latter impacts the patient's life. For example, anxiety might lead to many undesired consequences, one of which is recurrent emergency department visits. Other more grave concerns might include intentional hiding of symptoms. This is commonly seen in patients who have jobs that require employees to not have a condition that may put others at risk, such as airplane pilots.

PQRST

Having touched briefly on each of the above elements, we now have to explain a vital component of our practice, namely, is the progress note. Documentation in the form of a progress note serves many purposes: It should reflect that the elements above were thought of to ensure a comprehensive approach (think of your note as a thought organizer); it is a means to communicate with others; a note is our day-to-day patient's course diary to show the patient's trends; and the note may be used for medical legal, verification, or billing purposes.

The power of these black—or blue—words on white paper or screens is immense and should be recognized from the onset. With that in mind, descriptively speaking, a medical progress note should have qualitative elements that reflect the patient's input and our synthesis, and a quantitative element that should reflect the parameters we are monitoring to parallel the qualitative components.

For standardization purposes, several schemes have been developed for proper note writing. However, we propose utilizing the iAMOSMS scheme in Table 2 again with a minor modification as of day 2. This modification is to exclude any redundant components under the Morbidities and Support System sections. Alternatively, it is very important to expand the section related to organ-specific indicators in particular to answer how these indicators are changing. This will reflect the trend the patient is following and might impact prognosis or dictate a change in therapy. Similarly, the Systemic section may have to be slightly expanded to include urine output, for example. This will certainly vary from one patient to another.

To explain the above, consider a patient who was admitted with pneumonia and was placed on antibiotics and is on the regular floor. You come in and notice the patient's mental status is not satisfactory, as he is now more sleepy and his pulse oxymeter is reading 88% saturation on room air. Both parameters are in our scheme and reflect a change. Therefore, we need to intervene and introduce new therapies.

The final components of the medical note are the synthesis and team's input parts. Among all the parts of the note, the synthesis part is the most critical in terms of revealing the quality of a note. This is where your input is noted. To clarify, most of the preceding components can be labeled under data gathering. However, analyzing this data, synthesizing a conclusion that describes a situation analysis, and suggesting/performing an intervention and documenting it are our tasks, and all go under this section. Here is where proper implementation of the iAMOSMS scheme is highly needed, because from that, we will see the trend that describes the patient's response to therapy. Analyzing this trend and commenting as to whether it shows a favorable or unfavorable response reflects that we are aware of our patient's situation. Central to this is our previous knowledge of the natural course of the illness with therapy. This course/trend is the reference standard to which we will cross-compare our patient's trend. It is useful that the sections of the iAMOSMS scheme are expanded and detailed to ensure the inclusion of all metrics needed to monitor the trend of the patient's response to therapy.

For example, certain complications of an illness or resolution of certain abnormalities occur after a number of days. Formation of left ventricle thrombus after a myocardial infarction or resolution of pneumonia findings on a chest X-ray will not occur on day 2. Hence, knowing when these will occur and monitoring them if needed will ensure that we know what we are after and the patient is in safe hands.

For simplicity purposes, synthesis should include:

1. Cross-comparing our patient's progress trend to that which is expected (including monitoring for certain time related complications)
2. Commenting on our patient's trend (favorable versus unfavorable) relative to the reference standard.
3. Revisiting why an unfavorable trend is noted
4. Suggesting an intervention/ change in approach to ameliorate the unfavorable discrepancy and stabilize the patient

To properly perform all the above, we need every possible information we can get for better data gathering. Also, and not surprisingly, having more than one mind reflecting about the patient brings in more brain power. Therefore, consulting the nursing team that is taking care of this patient is a self-evident step. After all, the nurse in charge of the patient is the person performing the first data collection swipe. This nurse is not only on the front line to report major life-threatening changes (acute desaturation or change in mental status such as loss of consciousness) but can also provide more information depending on the nurse's experience and level of knowledge and interest. Here, it is a must to highlight that to get more out of this individual, acknowledgment of his/her role is a must. Should we fail to do that, we risk losing an important source of information and another helping power. This will be further explained in the section on creating a culture of successful healing. However, nurses and other members, including dietitians, physiotherapists, and family members, have a lot that they can offer.

A clear example of this is the importance of early ambulation and physiotherapy to prevent bedsores, which are dreadful complications of hospitalizations and can lead to infections, prolonged hospital stay, or death. Similarly, proper dietary intake ensures that the body is provided with what it needs to produce its armamentarium. Individuals with low albumin levels secondary to poor dietary intake may develop lower extremity edema, which has its own set of complications. Albumin-bound drugs will need their doses to be adjusted according to serum albumin level.

Along that line of thought, our encounter with the patient is at a time point where this individual may be passing through a detrimental illness that is significantly altering his/her personality or judgment. We will not be able to ascertain this without cross-checking with family members as to how the patient is at baseline outside the hospital. This is important information not only because it reflects a change that needs to be addressed, but also because should the patient be passing through a psychiatric state that is affecting his/her overall judgment capacity, then this patient is not the right person to consent to or decline procedures.

A strong example of the above can be observed in heart failure patients with severe pump dysfunction. This group has very decreased overall perfusion, including to the brain. These patients' mental status and psychiatric situation improve dramatically after inserting left ventricular assist devices; this finding does not merely come from personal anecdotes. Thus, we should be aware of this while requesting their informed consent. Getting a proper psychiatric assessment may be warranted at some point to ensure they have sound judgment.

Once all the above steps are performed, then the next day, or reassessment time, is simply a repetition of the cycle. The number of notes to be written and frequency of revisits vary with the patient's condition and how fast things are developing.

In conclusion, we hope that in this chapter, we have detailed how to utilize the figures below as best as possible. In doing so, we recurrently emphasize concepts from different chapters. This is mostly because of our aim to reflect that an encounter with a patient is a complete, tightly related encounter and not a fragmented one. Hence, it is important to adhere to all the steps above in a micro manner while keeping our eyes open to the overall global picture.

Table 2 iAMOSMS (illness, AGE, MENTAL, ORGAN, SYSTEMIC, MORBIDITIES/MEDICATIONS, SUPPORT SYSTEM) Scheme

Illness	Age (years)	Mental Status	Organ Specific indicators	Systemic						Morbidities & Medications	Support System
				BUN (mg/dl)/Cr (mg/dl)	SBP	oC	RR/HR	O2	Labs		
Pneumonia	45	Alert but cannot swallow (nausea)	Multilobar	20/1.5	120	39.5	24/110	92%	15,000 WBC	DM Type 1	Lives alone

Patient Variables

UTI	Disoriented			
Pancreatitis	65	Auto-immune	Oncology	Cannot get home nurse / Working child is care provider
Etc.		Poly-pharmacy	CHF	

Healing: INDEX

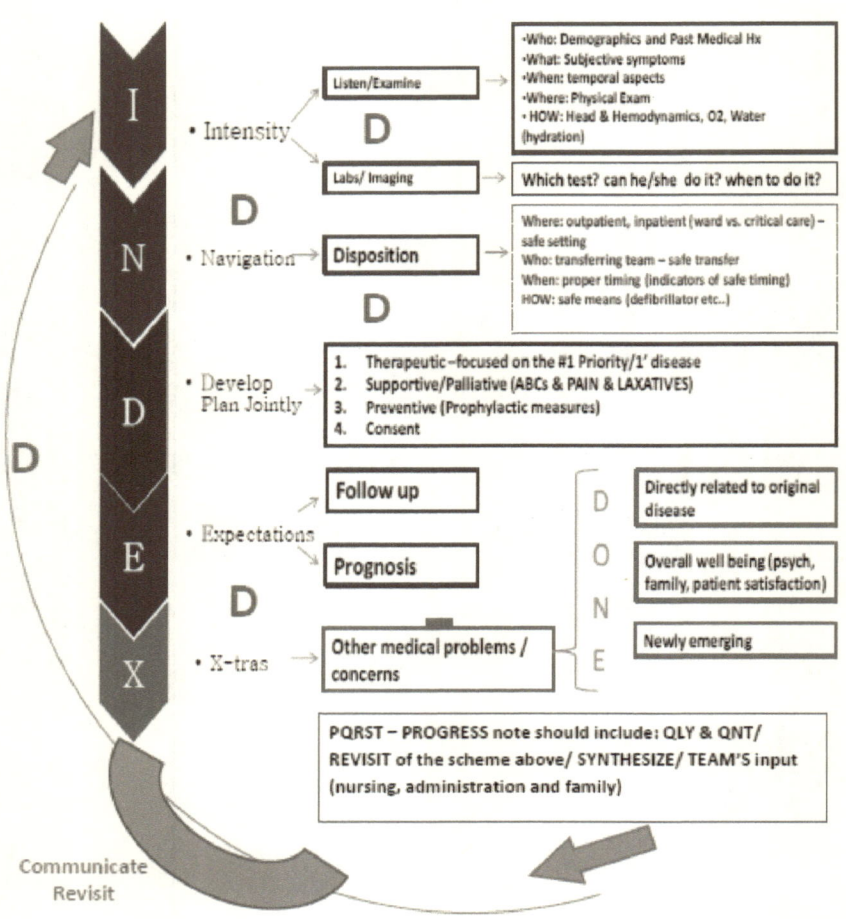

- Intensity
  - Listen/Examine → •Who: Demographics and Past Medical Hx
    - •What: Subjective symptoms
    - •When: temporal aspects
    - •Where: Physical Exam
    - • HOW: Head & Hemodynamics, O2, Water (hydration)
  - Labs/ Imaging → Which test? can he/she do it? when to do it?

D

- Navigation → Disposition → Where: outpatient, inpatient (ward vs. critical care) – safe setting
  - Who: transferring team – safe transfer
  - When: proper timing (indicators of safe timing)
  - HOW: safe means (defibrillator etc..)

D

- Develop Plan Jointly
  1. Therapeutic –focused on the #1 Priority/1' disease
  2. Supportive/Palliative (ABCs & PAIN & LAXATIVES)
  3. Preventive (Prophylactic measures)
  4. Consent

- Expectations
  - Follow up
  - Prognosis

D

- X-tras → Other medical problems / concerns

D O N E
- Directly related to original disease
- Overall well being (psych, family, patient satisfaction)
- Newly emerging

PQRST – PROGRESS note should include: QLY & QNT/ REVISIT of the scheme above/ SYNTHESIZE/ TEAM'S input (nursing, administration and family)

I N D E X

D

Communicate Revisit

The Universal Origin of the Ethics of Medical Practice

Hussain Isma'eel and Mohammad El-Obeidy

Today's world has shrunk because of the interconnectivity achieved by media, cheap traveling expenses, and migration of people (physicians and others). Therefore, it is neither uncommon nor surprising to find "dialogue space" enriched with discourse and dialectics about the transcultural differences in the implementation of ethics in medical practice. This is currently present (blogs, Facebook, etc.), was present since the days of Avicenna and even earlier, and will continue to be present. While this fact leads to healthy exchange, it strains our minds. This is more felt by practitioners who deal with individuals of different cultures or even find themselves practicing in a different culture altogether.

Hence, it is absolutely limited in our opinion to deal with health and sickness of humans with emphasis on the biology and lack of knowledge of the belief systems our patients hold. Conversely, patients should at some point be educated about the amount of mental discourse occurring in the mind of a physician while trying to guide the patients and respect their autonomy simultaneously. *Human-to-human interaction is fundamentally a bi-directionally influencing relationship.* Focusing on the commonalities and understanding and respecting the differences therefore becomes of prime importance. Ignoring these realities makes the physician–patient relationship deficient.

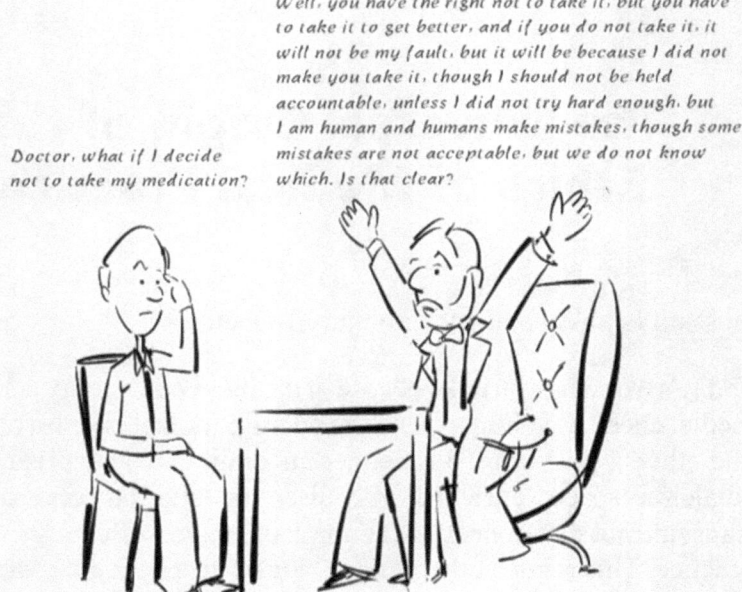

Illustration drawn by Dr. Fouad Boulos

That said, this chapter will introduce the three pillars of wise, balanced practice: 1. The worldly accepted fact: physicians are distinguished because of the role they chose to lead and should live up to; 2. The common universal ground for the four principles of ethics in clinical practice (autonomy, beneficence, nonmaleficence, and just/respectful approach to others) in various cultures; and 3. ....(these dots were left like this purposefully and will be filled in the last paragraph). For those who want the short answer, see Figure below.

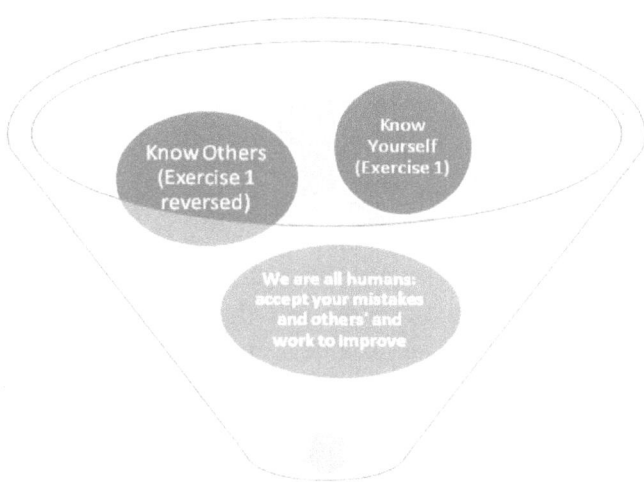

Whatever you wish that men would do to you, do so to them. (Ethics Course is Complete)

Pillar 1: Physicians are respected worldwide because of their role and they should live up to this.

Lifting and avoiding agony is among the most fundamental behaviors of all creatures. This is observed in animals and humans alike, but no doubt with varying degrees. In humans, however, as service exchange is far more advanced, some specialize in agony lifting (referred to as intervention from now onward). This statement is not in any way intended to undermine that the principle of prevention of agony occurrence (avoiding) also has its origins. Therefore, both functions of prevention and intervention are part of the services provided by physicians. Naturally, for prevention to exist, a preceding knowledge of the consequence of an ill-advised action must have been observed; this is called causality. Is it then not reasonable to deduce that those who are more diligent in recordkeeping and pattern recognizing would be more capable of guiding to prevent illness occurrence through ill-advised actions? Answering this question will lead to understanding the ladder of the levels of learning among the learners (one of the highest levels is that of the wise). The higher the level attained by this learner (wisdom), the more this learner will be sought after by those in need. This reflects the power of gravity of knowledge, which is literally and figuratively a power—the softest and kindest to which all creatures converge.

To illustrate, try to envision the wise men Hippocrates, Avicenna, Freud, Darwin, and Braunwald, among others. Ponder on these names and appreciate *how frequently* we refer to—or converge and link to their thoughts—these individuals. Only by doing so will you feel their gravity.

Now let it be clear that in our understanding, the above observation was restricted neither to a culture nor to a continent or a period of time. This is part of human nature and therefore universal. Denying this through attributing this to a certain culture is an unacceptable partiality. The oath of the Hindu physician, also known as the *Vaidya's oath*, was an oath taken by Hindu physicians and dates from the *fifteenth century BCE*. By inspecting its contents, we can clearly recognize the high expectations from a physician (this will be detailed further in the next paragraphs). *Assaf's oath* is a Jewish oath for physicians ascribed to Asaph ben Berechiahu, who lived between the *fourth to sixth century BC*. Similarly, the *Hippocratic oath* is an oath historically taken by those swearing to practice medicine in Ancient Greece. This oath dates back to the *fifth century BCE*, and it is an unneeded redundancy to highlight the reverence achieved by the holders of this oath, who had safe passage between countries—a universal passport that requires no entry visa. Moreover, the *Jewish Maimonides* considered, "The practice of medicine is an excellent way to develop the intellect and the character, and acquire knowledge of God, blessed be He. And when one becomes genuinely successful, his study and research are among the greatest types of service of God." *In Christianity, the Bible states*, "They that are healthy need not a physician but they that are sick." (Matt 9:12). Similarly, *in Islam,* the level of those who help heal is very highly revered *as is evident from the words of Allah*: "And if any one saved a life, It would be as if he saved the life of the whole people" (Quran 5:32), and from the words of the Prophet Mohammad (PBUH): "He who alleviates the suffering of a believer out of the sufferings of the world, Allah would alleviate his suffering from the sufferings of the Day of Resurrection, and he who finds relief for one who is hard pressed, Allah would make things easy for him in the Hereafter."

Having partly displayed the significance of physicians in history and in contemporary times, we suggest you then look within yourself and answer the following questions truthfully:

1. Have I felt this?
2. Have I recognized why others look up to me?
3. What were their expectations of me that I met that made them look up to me?

The answer to the second question is the one that this book is more interested in uncovering. One of the answers is: our code of ethics.

And the code of ethics is the subject of the following paragraphs.

In today's practice of medicine, and more so in the future, a universal code of common ethics is being pressed. While achieving the dissemination of this is probably possible, *variations on the implementation side of this code should be expected and accepted.* Actually, not accepting this contradicts the principle of autonomy in the universal code itself. Realistically, international applicability of a code is not an easy task. Physicians should take into consideration local cultural differences. It is this wisdom feature, and accepting and tolerating differences, that physicians now need to attain. Hence, this is the strain to our minds—as mentioned above—that we have to tolerate. Yes, what we recommend *may be* the sanest, but what the patient chooses is the sanest to him/her. And this is the core of patient-centered care: him/her.

To illustrate:

1. How many of us would have liked to call the last Muslim faithful terminal oncology patient "Do Not Resuscitate" but could not because of his/her belief?
2. How many of us would have just wanted to transfuse the last Jehovah's Witness patient to avoid the hypotension that occurred after surgery?
3. How many of us would have just wished that our Hindu/vegan patient ate meat or our Jewish patient ate nonkosher food instead of having to think about their dietary concerns?

Tolerance is a virtue we should live in accordance with. Have you not gotten depressed and desired to change people in the middle of such depression? Instead, find the common ground between their beliefs and yours so you can *better coach* and guide those who desire to change. (For further reading, we suggest "The Coach Approach").

Pillar 2: The UNIVERSAL common ground for the four principles of ethics in clinical practice (autonomy, beneficence, nonmaleficence, and just/respectful approach to others) in various cultures.

Here, we highlight the common ground for the four principles of ethics in clinical practice, namely, autonomy, beneficence, nonmaleficence, and justice/respectful approach to others, in several cultures.

Autonomy The concept of autonomy in ethics is probably among the most delicate to be approached. Modern Western medicine took the implementation side of this concept forward (over these last 40 years or so) to an extent that made it in possibly contradictory with other cultures some places. One of the implementation aspects of the concept of autonomy is informed consent. In our readings, the first clear order for informed consent that we could find goes back to Imam Ali Ibn Abi Taleb (PBUH) in Islam (seventh century AD) who stated, "All physicians and veterans, treating humans and animals, should take for themselves 'their innocence.' Otherwise, should they treat without taking their innocence and they harm, they are considered guarantors." Now this is one implementation aspect that just happened to be commonly present. This does not in any way suggest that other aspects will be shared. (However, it is interesting to note that the concept of malpractice insurance was also alluded to then.) In Chinese culture Chu Hui-ming (AD 1590) stated, "If the patient's prognosis was poor, the physician should say so at the very beginning so there would be no need to experience shame and reproach at the end." While this does not match in its clarity the informed consent that is recognized nowadays, this recommendation does state the need for clear communication of the situation and also that this clarity protects from reproach. Both elements are part of the consenting process we practice today and therefore approach its spirit.

If we are to rightfully admit to the fact that the current practice of autonomy is unique, then to look for the shared grounds for autonomy in culture, we should go back to the original question: *Are humans free in their choices?*

In line with the principle of autonomy, we choose to leave it to you to reflect on the statements below from each culture. We advise you to read more and discuss with the learned from each culture and develop your personal understanding. This is because this subject in particular is one that each culture below approaches in a more delicate manner than a simple statement cited in this book. Should we not recommend so, we would be self-contradictory, God forbid.

Judaism	Now the Lord God said, "Behold man has become like one of us, having the ability of knowing good and evil." (Genesis 3:22)
Islam	Certainly you are accountable for what you do. (Quran 16:93)
Christianity	It is for freedom that Christ has set us free. Stand firm, then, and do not let yourselves be burdened again by a yoke of slavery. (Galatians 5:1)
United Nations	You have the right to believe the things you want to believe, to have ideas about right and wrong, and to believe in any religion you want. (United Nations Human Rights Declaration (UNHRD) Article 18)
Chinese	It is man who makes the Tao great, not the other way around. (Confucius)
Indian	Now as a man is like this or like that, according as he acts, and according as he behaves, so will he be: a man of good acts will become good, a man of bad acts, bad. (Brihadaranyaka Upanishad 4.4.5-6)

Beneficence This refers to the tradition of acting in the patient's best interest. We find that this tradition and the others, except autonomy, are the most clearly stated universally. What is challenging, however, is the impartial implementation of this tradition when it contradicts the patient's autonomy.

For example:

Q1: What would you do if a relatively healthy and mentally intact 45-year-old lady prefers to treat a gangrenous cholecystitis at home using herbal medications?

On the other hand, an uncommonly faced difficulty in applying this is when we are challenged by cases where the patient cannot decide and others, family or else, are the decision makers. Here, would you be willing to overrule the decision of that other, whoever he/she is, and act based on beneficence?

For example:

Q2: What would you do if a two-year-old baby who is bleeding and hypotensive needs blood and the Jehovah's Witness parents are refusing the transfusion?

The answer to Q1 is: Respect the individual's belief.

The answer to Q2 is: Overrule the parents' decision and transfuse the baby.

Below is what each of the listed cultures promotes. Further explanation is needed to sharpen our understanding, for in practice we attain perfection.

Judaism   A beneficent soul will be abundantly gratified.—Talmud

Islam   And do good; indeed, Allah loves the doers of good. (Quran 2:195)

Christianity   Do not withhold good from those to whom it is due when it is in your power to do it. (Galatians 6:10)

United Nations All humans are endowed with reason and conscience, and should act toward one another in a spirit of brotherhood. (UNHRD Article 1)

Chinese   *The good physician* of the present day cherishes humaneness and righteousness . . . He cares not for vainglory, but is intent upon relieving suffering among all classes. He revives the dying and restores them to health: *his beneficence is equal to that of Providence.* (Kung Hsin in AD 1556)

Indian   After having finished your studies, with your medicaments *you shall assist* Brahmins, venerable persons, poor people, women, ascetics, pious people seeking your assistance, widows and orphans, and any one you meet on your errands *as if they were your own relatives.* This will be the right conduct. (Vaidya's oath)

Non-maleficence This refers to embracing the principle that we should not harm our patients neither through treatment nor research nor any other means. The most horrendous examples of maleficence in research are those that the Nazis performed on Jews and other Europeans. Nothing can justify this. Not even all the scientific information that was derived from these experiments is worth the pain of one individual in this process. No, the end does not justify the means. All the systems of beliefs listed below clearly state that as in Vaidya's Oath: You must put behind improper conduct.

Along the same line:

1. breaching confidentiality,
2. uncovering a patient beyond what is needed for examination for pride or lust,
3. denying a patient a second opinion because of egotism, greed, or falsehood,
4. delays in researching the best treatment out of sloth,
5. enforcing stringent visiting hours rules on a dying patient out of harshness, are all acts of maleficence that we should not indulge in.

All the cultures prohibit maleficence, so make sure to abide.

Judaism And what you hate, do not do to anyone. (Tobit 4.15)

Islam In Islam, there shall be no harm neither inflicted nor reciprocated. (Mohammad-PBUH)

Christianity Do not do evil that good may come. (Rom 12:21)

United Nations No one shall be subjected to torture or to cruel, inhuman or degrading treatment or punishment. (UNHRD Article 5)

Chinese Save life and do not kill any living creature. (Sun Szu-miao)

Indian Vaidya's Oath: You must put behind you desire, anger, greed, folly, pride, egotism, jealousy, harshness, calumny, falsehood, sloth, and improper conduct.

Justice   In seeking to maintain justice, physicians face several problems. Before explaining this principle further, we probably should share this story from the tradition. It is said that a mother was once asked, "Who among your children do you love the most? She replied, "The sick till he is well, the young and weak till he grows and becomes stronger, and the away till he comes back." Justice is learned from this. Justice is not only equality, but is also equity. And in equity, there is emphasis on priority (the sick till he is well is loved more). That said, physicians practicing public health or who are responsible for distributing resources need to emphasize the issue of numbers served.

For example:

1. An intervention can be covered by social security in certain countries if it is considered cost effective. We cannot expect a country that strives to combat malnutrition to reimburse heart assist devices. The current price of such a device can possibly treat several hundred malnourished children.

2. Some countries state it as a condition: Those older than 65 years have lesser chances of receiving transplantation.

The mechanism that oversees the development of the conditions above may appear to some as unjust. Here, remember that an impartial implementation of an unjust rule is just. Therefore, before questioning the end result of a process, learn the process, as you may end up agreeing to it or bettering it. Then, revisit the rule to avoid being among those who are the major losers, i.e., those who thought they were maintaining justice when they were not.

Similar to the principles of beneficence and nonmaleficence, the principle of justice is deeply rooted in all cultures as noted from the citations below.

Judaism   Blessed are they who maintain justice, who constantly do what is right. (Psalm 106:3)

Islam   And if you judge, judge between them with justice. Indeed, Allah loves those who act justly. (Quran 5:42)

Christianity	Do not pervert justice; do not show partiality to the poor or favoritism to the great, but judge your neighbor fairly. (Leviticus 19:15)
United Nations	In the exercise of his rights and freedoms, everyone shall be subject only to such limitations as are determined by law solely for the purpose of securing due recognition and respect for the rights and freedoms of others and of meeting the just requirements of morality, public order, and the general welfare in a democratic society. [UHHRD Article 29:(2)]
Chinese	If someone seeks help because of illness or on the ground of another difficulty, [a great physician] should not pay attention to status, wealth, or age, neither should he question whether the particular person is attractive or unattractive, whether he is an enemy or a friend, whether he is Chinese or a foreigner, or finally, whether he is uneducated or educated. He should meet everyone on equal ground. (Sun Szu-miao)
Indian	Assist Brahmins, venerable persons, poor people, women, ascetics, pious people seeking your assistance, widows and orphans, and any one you meet on your errands as if they were your own relatives. (Vaidya's oath)

Truthfulness and Respect for Others

Central to the adherence to the four principles above is adherence to truthfulness and respect for others. Otherwise, how can untrue statements be the source of maintaining justice? Or how can we preserve autonomy without respect for others?

Therefore, and with no redundancy, we provide the quotations that promote adherence to truthfulness and respect for others *universally*.

Truthfulness

Judaism   You shall not give a false testimony (Exodus 20: 12).

Islam   Allah doth command you to render back your trust to those to whom they are due. (Quran 4:58)

Christianity   Therefore, having put away falsehood, let each one of you speak the truth with his neighbor, for we are members one of another. (Ephesians 4:25)

United Nations

Chinese   Physicians should reflect on each case very conscientiously and should not engage in deceitful practice. If the patient's prognosis was poor, the physician should say so at the very beginning so there would be no need to experience shame and reproach at the end. [Chu Hui-ming (AD1590)]

Indian   Abandoning false speech . . . He speaks the truth, holds to the truth, is firm, reliable, no deceiver of the world . . . (The Samaññaphala Sutta)

Respect for others

Judaism   Did not He that made me in the womb make him also? – Talmud

Islam   Your creation and your resurrection will not be but as that of a single soul. Indeed, Allah is Hearing and Seeing. (Quran 31:28)

Christianity   Who desires all people to be saved and to come to the knowledge of the truth. (Timothy 2:4)

United Nations   All human beings are born free and equal in dignity and rights. (UNHRD Article 1)

| Chinese | He should look upon those who have come to grief as if he himself had been struck, and he should sympathize with them deep in his mind. Neither dangerous mountain passes nor the time of day, neither weather conditions nor hunger, thirst nor fatigue should keep him from helping wholeheartedly. (Sun Szu-miao) |
| Indian | Should even one's enemy arrive at the doorstep, he should be attended upon with respect. A tree does not withdraw its cooling shade even from the one who has come to cut it. – Mahabharata 12.146.5 |

Sources of confusion

Like all medical students, we also have to deal with confusing situations. As you noted in the sections above, the most important, if not the sole, cause of this confusion is when one principle is in opposition with another. Go back and read example 1 in the Beneficence section. You will note that this is an example where beneficence contradicts with autonomy. In this example we favored autonomy and respected the adult's decision because we opted that she is mentally intact to make a decision despite the fact it is most likely going to lead to unfavorable outcomes. Alternatively, in example 2 in this same section, we favored beneficence over autonomy because the baby's health could be seriously jeopardized because of a belief the parents hold and in which the baby has no say.

Take a deep breath here and accept that part of your role is the WISE.

We do acknowledge that in some instances, we may all feel frustrated with "wrong" decisions that patients make (example 1). However, it is important that you remember this is them and not you nor the medical practice. We should not be from those who feel great comfort with success (curing disease) and discomfort with failure to cure a disease. Our service transcends disease fighting; we are healers and therefore, we do not permit ourselves to adopt a false understanding that might lead us to feel discomfort with the profession at large. Should we do so, and we strongly discourage this understanding, then we will be the biggest losers.

Pillar 3: The central pillar

If you have reached this far, then you are ready for the third pillar—unless you have discovered it yourself. Pillar 3 simply states that we are humans and are hence insignificant by ourselves and significant as a limited tool for the Almighty to heal (a replaceable tool). Without us, his will will be completed, but if his will is exercised through us, then he has bestowed on to us a blessing. Count and cherish your blessings for you are in need for them to balance your nature. As humans, we are weak and vulnerable. As humans, we have an inclination to be hasty and to hoard. As humans, we have desires and weaknesses (sex, money, more knowledge, more power, laziness, more children, unchallenged opinions, better living conditions, etc.) As humans, we can do wrong, and the biggest losers are those who think they are doing right when they are doing wrong. As humans, we should comprehend that we need to be balanced in our understanding and our practice of our mission. From Pillar 3, recognize that

1. We are all subject to questioning and should surround ourselves at all times with those who question us. The loneliest person is he who thinks he is better than all.
2. We should recognize a problem and admit to it when we face one. The most delicate problem is that when two ethical principles seem contradictory (autonomy versus beneficence, beneficence versus nonmaleficence, or beneficence versus justice). Whenever you face such a situation, *consult those who are more knowledgeable and experienced than you. Do not act out of your interpretation,* and remember that there is always a first time to you, which is not the first time for another person.
3. We should act within our capabilities and surround ourselves at all times with those who motivate us to advance. The laziest is he who limits himself, and the cruelest is he who is cruel to himself.
4. We should know ourselves and our beliefs. Should our beliefs be in complete antagonism with that of our patient and hence

with our patient's requests, then do not hesitate to seek assistance or even refer this patient to another.

5. We should respect that in every act, we desire three shares: a divine share from God that he sees we are obeying him, an earthly share from the community that they see we are serving them, and a fair personal share for ourselves (fair compensation for our service, that we may at sometimes forego) so we know we have received a due and therefore nobody owes us anything more. A physician who denies these three desires is ignorantly denying his nature; and he who denies himself from receiving those in a balanced manner is ignorantly denying himself the opportunity to be protected from succumbing to a bad inclination at a vulnerable moment.

With this understanding, the circle is complete, and within this circle is you. Enlarge this circle while understanding it remains only a dot that is relative to the Infinite. Accept and practice your role, and the Infinite will appease you, and you will be appeased at the Infinite.

Exercise 1A

Step 1: Answer the questions below

The purpose of this step is to maximize your insight and see how others see you, i.e., your image. View the figure below, as we will go back to it after the exercise).

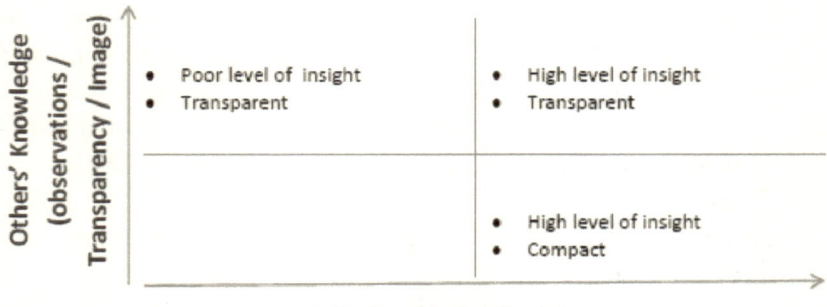

If you answer yes to any of them, acknowledge that you are imperfect. Know that you have breached your oath and your commitment is under question. But more importantly,

1. keep your answers to yourself for now;
2. discuss them with a mentor;
3. know that we all may answer yes to some of them;
4. some of us admit to it while others do not. What is important is that you know and are honest to yourself;
5. keep an open and merciful eye when you see a yes in others;
6. do not accept a yes in you or another, but instead, seek the background that led to it; you may be surprised to have misperceived things; and
7. be merciful and very cautious in your opinion for we are all under observation.

Use your experience in the wards to answer these and be honest with yourself.

Do not answer these questions if you have not had at least one year of experience in the wards. You will know yourself better once you have practice and have been tempted—not in theory.

Step 2: Should you answer yes to any of the following, seek help early on by discussing this with your mentor.

Step 3: *You can also get a very trusted colleague to answer these questions for you by replacing "Do you" in the questions with "Do you know if Mr./Ms. has done this?"* Do not share with him your answers. This is a step that takes a lot of bonding and trust. You may be able to do it later. There are things to share and others not to be shared.

Step 4: Take your answers and match them with those you received from your colleague and friend.

Step 5: Now refer to the figure below to match your replies with those you got from your friend:

A. What you and your friend said yes to is an undesired trait that you know of and is known to him/her. Try to fix it as what is known to your friend and forgiven by him/her may not be forgiven by another.

B. What you said yes to and your friend said no to is an undesired trait that you have but is unknown to him/her. Try to fix it before it becomes known so your image is not tarnished.

C. What you said no to and your friend said yes to is an undesired trait that indicates a possible mismatch between your insight and image. Refer to step 6.

D. What you and your friend said no to are oath-breaching features that you have not committed. You should be graceful that you have not fallen.

Step 6: Take elements of mismatch (C) and discuss them with your friend. Ask your friend to provide you with a real example for each mismatch. If the friend is unable to do so, then the friend should be able to admit that it is not true, and therefore should change his/her perception of you. Alternatively, if an example is provided, then you should be ready to accept it and work on it.

Friend's Replies are the closest to your Image:

	Yes	No
Yes	• Matched • Recognize others see you and your mistakes • If you see their mistakes, be merciful	• Your fault is not known • Be grateful for having a better image • Work on preserving this through avoiding this mistake
No	• Your image is worse than what you think • Discuss with your friend • If this is a defect, add it to the yes/yes list • If not true, be grateful for the opportunity to correct your image, and add it to the No/No category	• Be grateful that you have not committed this yet • Be grateful that your image is not tarnished with this

(Left vertical axis label: Your replies correspond to your insight:)

Remind yourself: those younger have done less mistakes, and those older have done more good

If you fail to do so now, this may be your weakness in the future.

The most troubling falls are those that could have been dealt with at an earlier stage.

Exercise 1: Oath commitment insight/image matching questions

		Yes		Comment on your answer:
1-	Do you (do you know of someone who) smile more to the rich than the poor?	Me	Another	
2-	Do you give more time to the rich than the poor?	Me	Another	
3-	Do you give preferential treatment to people in powerful positions?	Me	Another	

4- Do you imitate out of fun or ridicule a patient you have seen? Me   Another

5- Do you fantasize about a patient? Me   Another

6- Do you favor a patient over another because someone spoke on behalf of the other? Me   Another

7- Do you speak of a colleague's mistake without aiming to correct it for him? Me   Another

8- Do you prescribe a medication because of a relationship with the medical representative? Me   Another

9- Do you prescribe a medication because of a relationship with the pharmaceutical industry? Me   Another

10- Do you favor patients based on their gender? Me   Another

11- Do you look at a patient with lust?   Another

12- Do you uncover the patient beyond what is needed? Me   Another

13- Do you preferentially order a test from which you gain income instead of another test? Me   Another

14- Do you not seek assistance in a medical case that challenged you because of egotism? Me   Another

15- Are you lazily not working on researching the best treatment for the patient?   Me   Another

16- Are you lazy to reply to a patient's call or to attend to your pager?   Me   Another

17- Do you or do you know of someone who does not empathize with a patient's pain and does not provide adequate analgesia?   Me   Another

18- Do you speak harshly to patients?   Me   Another

19- Do you speak harshly about patients?   Me   Another

20- Do you or do you know of someone who speaks about patients in a public place (such as elevators)?   Me   Another

21- Do you or do you know of someone who writes on the medical note what was not done (physical exam, etc.)?   Me   Another

22- Do you plan to leave early and keep work for colleagues that should have been attended to earlier?   Me   Another

23- Do you wrongfully reduce the time given to a patient to increase the clinic's capacity?   Me   Another

24- Do you reduce the effort, quality, and time of a procedure to meet another goal at the expense of a patient?   Me   Another

25- Do you or do you know of someone who permits himself or his students to learn on patients despite the patient's pain?   Me   Another

26- Do you not disclose to the patient all risks from a procedure because you stand to gain something (educational or money)?   Me   Another

27- Do you overinflate the risk of a procedure to avoid doing what you are incapable of and do not refer the patient to a doctor who is more capable?   Me   Another

28- Do you disrespect the will of a mentally intact patient because you think that as a doctor, you know better?   Me   Another

29- Do you go with the family's desire and not protect the patient's best interests to avoid trouble with the family?   Me   Another

30- Do you hide a mistake that caused a problem to the patient and do not admit it to the responsible body?   Me   Another

31- Do you avoid standing for the patient's best interest out of fear of repercussions from an administrator?   Me   Another

32- Do you provide false promises about a treatment (in oncology, for example)?   Me   Another

33-	Do you not provide the prognosis after therapy for a patient (also in oncology for example)?	Me	Another
34-	Do you in the name of serving many compromise the service of one of those (to increase bed turnover rate for example)?	Me	Another
35-	Do you or do you know of someone.........(add your list)	Me	Another

Exercise 1B: Get to know others' commitment to the Oath, i.e., your institution's culture

Step 1: Answer the questions above about some of the people around you, particularly those in key positions.

Step 2: Realize that some of your answers may be real, and others may not match the reality.

Step 3: Be ready to deal with these realities (accept this culture and work on yourself to improve and do not allow yourself to be influenced negatively). This is the top priority; the others are important, but not as important as you not committing the mistakes others do. Each is responsible for his/her mistakes first. Correcting for others is another step that is important but has its pathways also.

Professionalism - Many definitions of professionalism are given. Ours is very simple: *Professionalism is applied ethics* (ethical behavior). This can be summarized by applying the Golden Rule: Whatever you wish that men would do to you, do so to them. (*Matthew 7.12*).

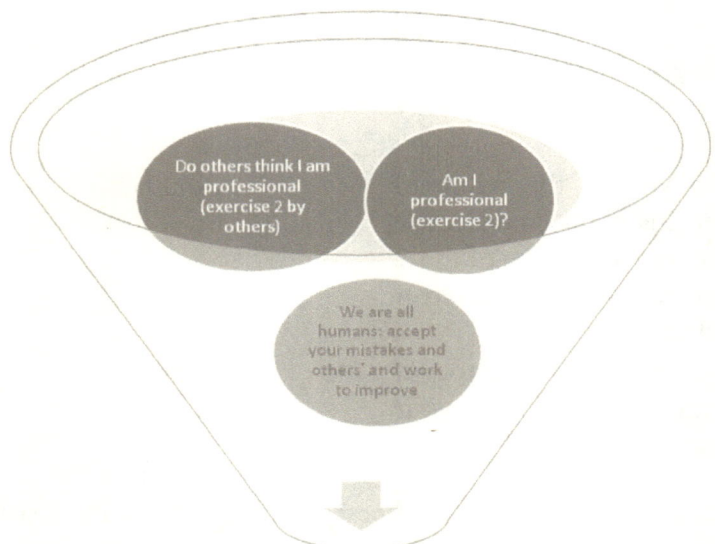

Professionalism is APPLIED Ethics. Whatever you wish that men would do to you, do so to them. (Ethics 001)

Therefore, and to avoid redundancy, after sitting for Exercises 1A and 1B, sit for *Exercise 2.*

Exercise 2

1.   Answer the questions below to yourself.
2.   Ask a colleague and a senior resident to answer these for you. (You can ask some of those in the circles below to answer the same questions for you, but this is a more advanced step that is important for the institution's culture. We leave it to you to decide.)

Responsibility

- Do I sometimes fail to follow through on tasks?
- Do I sometimes fail to arrive on time?
- Do I sometimes fail to accept blame for failure?

Maturity

- Do I sometimes make inappropriate demands?
- Am I sometimes abusive and critical at times of stress?

- Do I sometimes fail to listen well?

Communication skills

- Am I sometimes hostile?
- Am I sometimes deprecating to others?
- Am I sometimes sarcastic?
- Am I sometimes loud or disruptive?
- Do I sometimes breach patient confidentiality?

Respectful

- Do I sometimes appear insensitive to the physical and emotional needs of others?
- Do you see me as biased or discriminatory?

External appearance

- Does the way I dress sometimes appear to be discordant with my job as a physician?
- Does the way I look (shaved, tidy, etc.) sometimes appear to be discordant with my job as a physician?

3. Compare your answers with those of others.
4. Those that do not match need to be discussed and addressed.
5. This is the area that needs improvement. Work on it.

Start by self-observance then get external verification to validate your conclusions.

This is what we mean by "We are all under observation."

Here:

1. Beware who you ask to fill this out for you. You do not want your input to be tarnished by biased individuals.
2. It is preferable that you always rely on trustworthy colleagues and seniors.
3. There are cultural variations, and therefore the range of normal behavior varies.

4.   Your objective is to stay within the center and not on the extremes. Being balanced is being near the center of gravity; being balanced does not mean at the middle.

It is important to ensure that what we think of ourselves is aligned with how the majority of the others see us. *This is INSIGHT to project our IMAGE.* There are several reasons for a mismatch between your image and what you know about yourself. Strive to appear ethical and professional; your image and internal values positively feed onto each other, so work on both. Remember: "When there is no human to see me, I see myself."

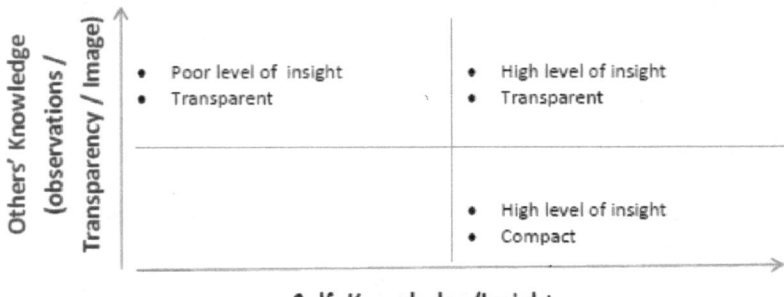

Self- Knowledge/Insight

Last: *Do not worry. We all have our defects.*

I personally have many.

Manage yours early on, and combat self-conceit.

As a hint for a future exercise, try to figure out: *What is self-conceit?* It is within the answers we will get from the above.

More importantly, this exercise needs to be repeated after several years. We tend to change over time, so make sure you change for the better!

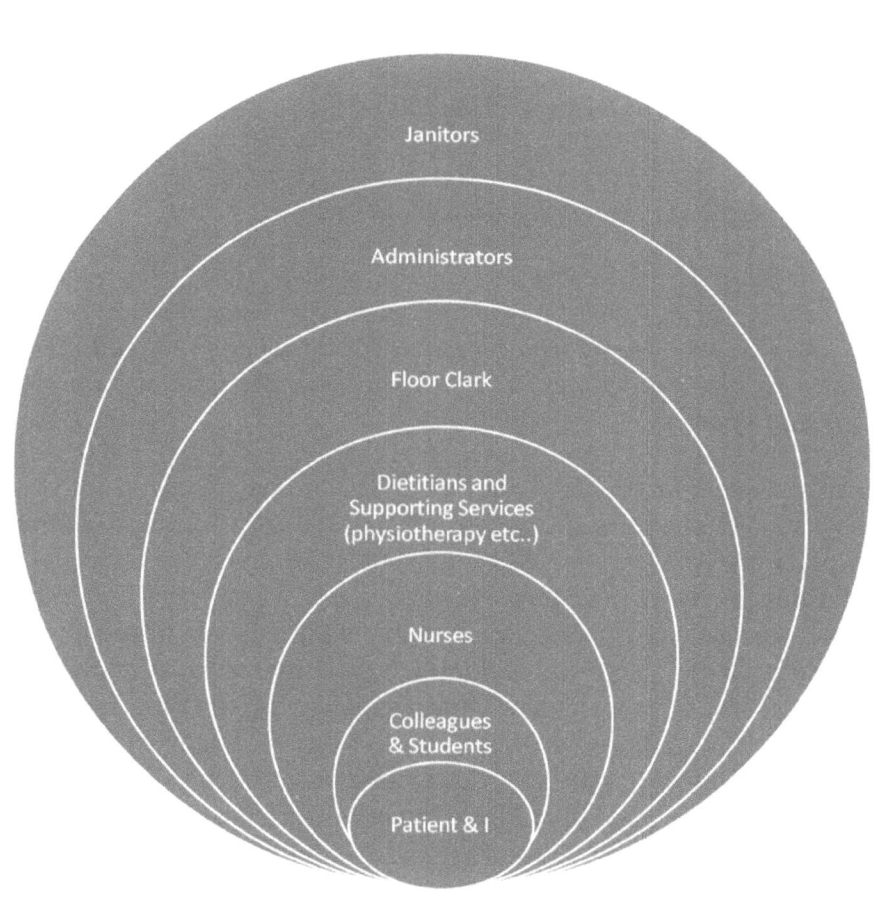

Janitors

Administrators

Floor Clark

Dietitians and
Supporting Services
(physiotherapy etc..)

Nurses

Colleagues
& Students

Patient & I

Choosing Your Specialty: A Process that Begins with YOU

Hussain Isma'eel and Fatima Ghaddar

An insightful medical student once told me:

"By the time I figured out what was expected of me as a medical student in any rotation, I would have already approached the end of it. And this was when I would realize that I had not had the time to really absorb and reflect on whether this was the specialty I really wanted to pursue."

Throughout your medical journey, this feeling of uncertainty is very common and is also very normal at many times. And this is probably what makes choosing your specialty among the most straining processes that you could go through. It is one decision whose repercussions you would bear for years. Is this starting to sound like a decision for a long-term relationship? Well, in many ways, it is. It is a relationship from which you expect satisfaction, whether financial, intellectual, or otherwise. Hence, when your chosen specialty does not fulfill your expectations, you can be prone to frustration. That is why it is very important to know where you are heading before you decide on one.

The gist from this chapter is as follows:

1. Know yourself.
2. Research the intended specialty and seek maximal know-how (i.e., facts) about it.
3. Perform a matching linkage between your preferences and the characteristics of the intended specialty.

4. Explore paramedic and non-clinical options. Remember that your medical degree is a doorway to more than clinical practice.

5. Do not settle for a choice that is just "not so bad;" under stress, a choice that was initially "not so bad" can become unbearable.

6. Remember to be passionate about your chosen specialty; passion is your truest guarantee for better future! After all, at this point in your career, all your career choices lie between the good and the better. You will have to make a huge, fundamental mistake to really bring yourself down. So you might as well choose a path that you really like and are comfortable with ☺.

7. Do not let some transient phase of exhaustion from previous years of your medical education dictate your long-term career choices. Relax, reflect, and take your time!

During your undergraduate medical education, you are simultaneously studying medicine, clinical skills, epidemiology, biostatistics, communication skills, health administration, bioethics, and professionalism, in addition to learning how to apply these disciplines in the context of multilayered organizations of which you are just one layer. Given the multiple levels of learning that you are going through, it is only natural to feel overwhelmed and off-balance. Such frustration can distort your perceptions about certain specialties and, therefore, can affect your decisions about them. That is why it is very important to identify and label your feelings (whether positive or negative) during a certain rotation. However, these feelings are only a reflection of that particular experience and, therefore, may or may not be extrapolated. That is why it is also important to seek widely accepted facts about a specialty. One of this chapter's goals is to help you make informed decisions about long-term career choices by identifying your feelings, getting facts about a certain specialty, and finally linking your feelings to the correct trigger, which, by the way, may or may not be related to the specialty you are considering.

You will note that in the coming sections, I will put a lot of emphasis on emotions. This is because emotional intelligence is very important in any decision making process. According to Daniel Goleman, author of the groundbreaking book Emotional Intelligence: Why it Can Matter More than IQ, the root of the word emotion is motere, the Latin verb "to move," and the prefix "e" denotes "move away." This means that there is a tendency to move in every emotion. And to make sure that you are moving in the right direction, i.e., toward a better career choice, it is very relevant to understand your emotions and to link them to their causes. You do not want to be deterred from an appropriate career choice just because a faculty member or one house staff whom you rotated with made your life a living hell. (I highly recommend further reading about emotions, decision-making, and emotional intelligence).

To make my recommendations easier to digest, I will be structuring them into the following steps:

Step 1: Identifying your emotions

The first step in your decision making process is to identify the emotions and perceptions that you develop toward the experiences you go through in medical school (for the sake of this chapter, I will be referring to your clinical rotations as your primary experiences, because they are very likely to influence your career decisions).

Are these emotions positive? Are they negative? To help you determine that, I have collated the following 17 questions that you can ask yourself as you reflect on your experience in any of your rotations:

1. During this rotation, have I felt insignificant and replaceable?
2. During this rotation, have I felt that my contributions are not needed nor appreciated?
3. During this rotation, have I felt that I was mostly required to do the paperwork?

4. During this rotation, have I felt that the residents who were teaching me were disrespectful to me or disrespectful in general?

5. During this rotation, have I felt that there was no one I could look up to as a role model?

6. During this rotation, have I felt intimidated by a faculty member?

7. During this rotation, have I felt intimidated by the fact that my inexperience could have led to a problem in patient care?

8. During this rotation, have I felt that I was not well supported (educationally or mentoring wise)?

9. During this rotation, have I felt that there was not enough use of technology and there was more that could have been done for the patient?

10. During this rotation, have I felt that there was a need to listen more to patients and this was not something I was willing to do?

11. During this rotation, have I felt that the patients tended to be less respectful of faculty members compared with other rotations?

12. During this rotation, have I felt that the nurses tended to be less respectful of the house staff or faculty members compared with other rotations?

13. During this rotation, have I felt that the nurses tended to be intimidated by the house staff or faculty members compared with other rotations?

14. During this rotation, have I felt that the working hours were longer and more demanding compared with other rotations?

15. During this rotation, have I felt overburdened with personal issues (e.g., family problems, partner problems, illness, financial challenges, etc.)?

16. During this rotation, have I felt that the patients' complaints were difficult to attend to?

17. During this rotation, have I felt that the patients were very sick and were anticipated to have poor outcomes (e.g., death) more frequently than in other rotations?

If you answer yes to any of the above questions, this indicates that you have developed a negatively charged emotion from a particular rotation. Now, to identify positive feelings you have had about a particular rotation, repeat the above questions but in a positive light. If you answer yes to any of the "positively transformed" questions, this indicates that you have developed a positively charged emotion from a particular rotation.

In general, human beings tend to sway away from experiences that generate in them negatively charged emotions, and they tend to seek those that generate positively charged ones. Keep this notion in mind for now as I will be getting back to it once I reach step 3.

Step 2: Seeking facts about a specialty

By now, you would have identified your emotions toward a certain rotation. But this is not enough! To complete your full understanding of your emotions, you will need to seek facts about that particular specialty, regardless of your own emotions.

But how can you research a specialty of interest? What criteria can you follow to make sure you have covered all the facts? To do that, check Table 1 below, in which I propose some criteria/features to look at when researching a certain specialty.

Potential Criteria for Consideration in a Specialty	Food for Thought
Type of specialty: surgical *versus* medical	• The biggest misconception is that good surgeons are not good internists. Adequate patient care inside the hospital postoperatively is instrumental for adequate patient outcomes. If surgeons are not good at this, then the patients' outcomes will be poor. • Some societies are more inclined to value surgeons more than prevention specialists. Identify which society you live in and whether or not you yourself believe that or not.

Age of patients: pediatrics/ adults/ geriatrics	1. Can you deal with families of patients in general? 2. Can you deal with moms? 3. Can you deal with demented patients? 4. Can you deal with the demented patients' families? 5. Can you deal with/perform procedures on babies? 6. Can you deal with end-of-life care issues?
Type of management: Acute management (ED, critical care)	▪ Specialties that rely on acute management require prompt decision making. ▪ Stress tolerance has to be high in these specialties. ▪ Answer the professionalism exercise, and reflect on how you behave under stress in other situations.
Type of management: Chronic management	1. Chronic diseases, such as COPD, CAD, and rheumatological diseases in general, are more suited to an outpatient setting 2. They require motivational communication skills and a lot of patience.
Setting of encounters: Outpatient *versus* inpatient; High *versus* minimal/no patient contact (radiology or pathology)	▪ Try to see if you are more of a people person (not only what you like but also whether others see you like this). Minimal or no patient contact specialties include pathology and laboratory medicine, and diagnostic radiology (NB: Interventional radiology is different).

Working hours	<ul><li>ED shifts have more or less fixed working hours.</li><li>Pathology/radiation therapy are also fixed.</li><li>Critical care specialties are more variable as far as working hours are concerned.</li></ul>
Use of technology	<ul><li>In technology-driven specialties, you need to stay up to date.</li><li>Only a few sites will be willing to pay for continuous upgrade of their technology. Keep this in mind.</li><li>Robotic technologies are not widely prevalent yet. Also, if you are an imaging specialist, you can only function in the institution in which this machine is present (note how widely spread ultrasound machines are compared with MRIs, for example).</li></ul>
Use of interventions and procedures	<ul><li>This is shared between surgery and interventional cardiology, interventional radiology, interventional gastroenterology, etc.</li><li>You have to be gifted with your hands.</li><li>If you are not, you need practice, which needs volume. If you do not practice enough, you will be a mediocre interventional physician.</li></ul>

Income (intervention and procedure-based *versus* patient volume-based- clinic)	■ The income subject is a subject that you have to look into objectively and rationally (this will be dealt with in a separate section in this chapter). ■ Example: Interventional gastroenterologists (ERCP, EUS biopsies, etc.) *versus* endoscopies alone. ■ Similarly, think of other specialties; endocrinology, for example, is patient volume based.
Workplace setting: Academic institutions *versus* private practice	1. Get the criteria of promotion of an academic faculty member to have an idea of your potential responsibilities 2. Compare the financial returns of both paths and whether the difference matters to you.
Specialties that involve reproductive and/ or excretory organs (obstetrics and gynecology/urology)	1. Go through the list of the diseases these specialties treat and put a % on the number of cases that a generalist sees and figure out if you can spend that much of your time dealing with these cases. Of course, if you sub-specialize, that will shift the %s.
Special topic: Dealing with death: common *versus* rare occurrence, acute/sudden *versus* expected occurrence etc.	2. Try to assess your ability and tolerance in dealing with death.

Table 1 Criteria to consider when seeking facts about a specialty

Step 3: Linking your emotions to facts about a specialty

At this point of your thinking process, you know the emotions you developed in a rotation, and you have collected the necessary facts about a certain specialty. What do you do with this information?

Figure 1 shows a proposed algorithm to help you cross-tabulate your positive and negative perceptions of a specialty against the facts that you collected about the specialty.

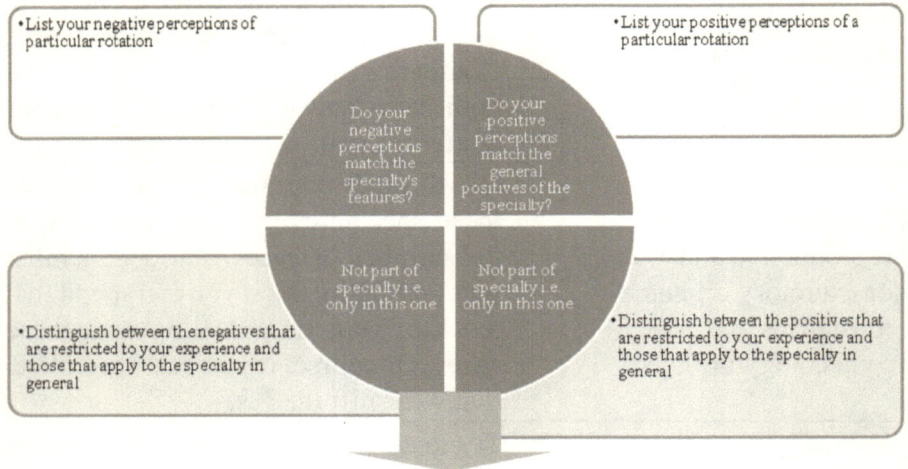

• List your negative perceptions of particular rotation

• List your positive perceptions of a particular rotation

Do your negative perceptions match the specialty's features?

Do your positive perceptions match the general positives of the specialty?

Not part of specialty i.e. only in this one

Not part of specialty i.e. only in this one

• Distinguish between the negatives that are restricted to your experience and those that apply to the specialty in general

• Distinguish between the positives that are restricted to your experience and those that apply to the specialty in general

		Your Perceptions of this Rotation/Specialty	
		Positive Perceptions	Negative Perceptions
Specialty Features and Facts	True	• Here lie the true positives; the features of this specialty fit you. • This is where you want to be.	• Here lies a mismatch, i.e., this rotation *triggered negativity that is inherent to the specialty itself.* • These feelings are highly likely to recur should you choose this specialty.
	False	• Here lies a mismatch, i.e., this *rotation triggered positivity that is not truly inherent to the specialty* (maybe it was the effect of the hospital setting, faculty members, etc.) • These positive feelings may or may not recur in other situations	• Here lie the false negatives, i.e., this rotation triggered negativity that is not inherent to the specialty itself. • Do not permit these feelings to sway you from this specialty.

In a nutshell:

- **You need to aim to be in the TRUE/POSITIVE box because you can function best over there and distinguish yourself.**
- **Do not mislead yourself by going elsewhere.**

Figure 1. Cross-tabulation of emotions and facts regarding a specialty

The true/positives box is where you fit, i.e., in the specialty that gives you the most positive feelings that are truly part of that specialty. To be very realistic, it will not be surprising that the individuals in that specialty will be closer to your personality as they probably worked out things in a way similar to how you just did ☺.

You may ask why this cross-tabulation is necessary. As I previously mentioned, human beings tend to shy away from negatively charged experiences and seek positively charged ones. If this tendency is not regulated, it can underlie a real risk because it can blind one's judgment. So even though it is important to acknowledge one's emotions, it is just as important not to falsely attribute one's emotions to the wrong trigger. No one wants to choose to be deterred from a specialty because he/she looked up or down on a faculty member in that specialty, was experiencing difficult personal problems, or simply worked with negative colleagues.

The following are real-life examples of medical students whose emotions blurred their perceptions of certain specialties:

Example 1: The nursery intensive care unit (NICU) experience

There was this medical student who hated the NICU rotation. He did not know why he was very emotionally negative about it. It took him a while to figure out that he needed regular daylight and that the number of hours he spent inside the unit, in which blue lights are used to treat hyper-bilirubinemia, had affected his mood so negatively that it affected his perception of the whole experience all together.

This realization was an important turning point in his decision making process because it helped him to identify the real trigger of his negative emotions and therefore allowed him to ask himself the right questions. Some of these questions included "Are all NICUs void of sunlight?" "If not, should I be working in one with some sunlight, or should I be taking breaks during the day to get some sun?"

It is important to avoid the confusion that this medical student went through (who, by the way, in response to his impulsive emotions came close to quitting medicine, divorcing, and even abandoning his religious faith! But that's another story.).

Example 2: Being on the verge of quitting (whether professionally or personally)

When does someone consider quitting? Quitting a job, for example? It is basically when you reach the edge of a cliff, i.e., when you lose your belief in that job. It is similar to when you decide to get a divorce, i.e., when you lose your belief in sustaining the relationship. You can even extrapolate the same chain of questions when assessing your relationship with God or nature or anything you believe in.

Let me start with the marriage example. If you feel in your marriage that you are no longer capable of managing conflicts and that the only time you feel secure is when good things are happening, then you know you are sitting on the edge of a cliff. Before you get to this point, follow the recipe below.

Number 1: Recognize that you are on the edge of a cliff.

Number 2: Take a step back, and consider whether you have done enough. For example, rather than running away, consider investing in your marriage by infusing love in your relationship or by compromising. Such initiatives can take you off the cliff to safer ground and can help you make clearer decisions.

As for the example related to your job, the situation is similar. If you feel in your job that you are no longer capable of managing conflicts and that the only time you feel secure is when good things are happening, again, you know that you are sitting on the edge of a cliff. Here is some advice to avoid hasty decisions to quit.

Number 1: Recognize that you are on the edge of a cliff.

Number 2: Take a vacation and revisit/seek help to try to understand what drove you to the cliff. You may be surprised when you realize that your perceptions may be misleading you. After all, your perceptions are the result of your interpretations of situations and your own inclinations. That is why it is essential to question why you are feeling a certain way and to keep in check with how things are heading. Thinking out loud with a wise friend or seeking the advice of a mentor can help sometimes in this process of figuring out how to achieve your goals and to understand how your perceptions are affecting your decisions.

My takeaway message from the above examples is the following: Reaching the edge of a cliff without realizing how you got there can jeopardize a relationship or can cost you a career sometimes. Taking serious steps to stay in check can help you avoid reactive behaviors and immature decisions. It can also help you grow more insight into your own vulnerability as a human being and the manifestation of that vulnerability in different aspects of your life, whether it relates to your career, friendships, family and intimate relationships, or even your relationship with God.

Step 4: Doing it yourself

Knowing steps 1 through 3 is not enough. It is essential that you practice them yourself.

1. Plug in all the negative feelings you answered to the 17 questions into Figure 1.
2. Plug in the positive feelings into Figure 1 as well.
3. If you want to add more questions to the list above, please feel free to do so; this is your opportunity to bring it all out on the table.
4. Research the specialties you are considering based on the criteria proposed in Table 1. Even though Table 1 contains a lot of validated elements, it is in no way comprehensive, so feel free to add parameters as you see fit.
5. Return to Figure 1 to plug in the specialty facts and to do the proper linkages.
6. Validate what you have done with one and, more preferably, more than one specialist in the field. Try to get the opinion of both junior and senior professionals who are successful in the field you researched.
7. Proceed to identify what the true/positives are.

Step 5: What about alternatives to clinical practice?

Before proceeding with your thought process, take a step back and consider the following questions (these are questions that are rarely spoken about throughout your medical training):

1. Do you really want to go for a clinical training?
2. Are there options in the medical profession other than clinical practice?

It is pivotal to understand that your medical degree is way more than just a license to treat patients. It is so far the highest attainable degree certifying that you have acquired a foundation of scientific knowledge in human health. There are various tracks that can branch out from mainstream medicine, such as the following:

1. Clinical tracks
2. Research tracks such as physician scientists tracks, as in the case of professionals who pursue MD/PhD degrees or master's degrees in the basic sciences such as biology, physiology, and biochemistry.
3. Public health tracks that include healthcare management, health promotion, and health epidemiology, and include work in nongovernmental organizations (work in these organizations can be clinically and/or public health related, as in the case of Doctors Without Borders)
4. Educational tracks (e.g., medical education)
5. Business tracks (e.g., careers in the pharmaceutical industry or in social entrepreneurship)
6. Interdisciplinary tracks as in health professionals who pursue higher education in disciplines outside of the health profession, such as engineering, bioinformatics, artificial intelligence, and law

Engaging in a reflective process that includes these non-clinical options will enable you to make more informed choices about your future career. By following the same logic in Figure 1, you can get the facts about these paramedical career options and match them with your preferences and capabilities.

Step 6: Thinking about the logistics

So when should you start engaging in this thinking process and how? You need to make time for this in your busy schedule because it is the most important step that will dictate your future career.

To save time, one way of going about researching different specialties is by doing it in groups, i.e., with other medical students. Each group member can compile facts for one or two specialties and upload them on a shared folder so that the whole group can benefit from them and save time. By the time the Med 4 year is over, together you may have covered numerous specialties—far more than if each one of you worked alone. Also, by working together, you can benefit from one another's perspectives.

Also, you may want to consider taking one year after your Med 4 graduation just for experimentation and exploration or with a light load. Do not be concerned about wasting a year, because in medicine, the sooner you worry less about the time factor—particularly in this stage—the better your outcome will be.

Other logistic elements to consider are where you want to do your training (in your country, abroad, etc.) and where you can find a good training program. These issues need researching too. I will not be dwelling on them in this chapter. However, they are important to think about.

Step 7: Staying realistic about the money

Thinking early about money is necessary because it has a huge bearing on your future feelings or emotions. In today's economy and the declining trust in physicians, you are encouraged to approach the financial aspect of medicine with a realistic attitude.

Before I elaborate further, consider the following example:

The Med 4 Post-training Vision

During a rotation with my medical students, I engaged them in an exercise to help them match their financial expectations with their potential career choices. One of the medical students, who was not in a relationship at the time, volunteered for the exercise. I started by asking him, "How do you envision yourself living after completing your training? Paint the picture and list the items you desire with a timeline if possible." He proceeded by sharing how much he cared about having the following elements shortly after completing his specialization:

Elements of his vision	# of years attained postspecialization	Cost in USD
1. Buy a fancy sports car	1	
2. Buy a spacious apartment in one of the high-end areas in his country	2	
3. Get married and hold a really extravagant ceremony	1–3	

Table 2 Elements, timeline, and cost of a career vision

Before he continued listing his items, I asked him to approximate the cost of each item in his vision. After that, I asked him to open up the Doctor's Annual Pay reference on the Internet from one of the resources and calculate his projected income after removing the taxes. By going through one item after the other, this individual recognized that he was being unrealistic. Who knows? Maybe he had been lured into the saying, "Our happiness is measured by how much we can consume." By intending to consume way beyond his income, this individual was either setting himself up for disappointments or bank loans.

What was even more alarming in this individual's thought process was the timeline that he has set for himself and how he did not carefully integrate his own social context. What I mean is the following: This individual comes from a rather conservative religious background, and he was not willing to consider premarital relationships. At the same time, he was not willing to get engaged or married before buying *the apartment and car! As you can tell, this individual had cornered himself in a situation that was going to keep him sexually frustrated for quite some time.*

To avoid falling into the same trap, ask yourself the following questions:

1. What are the financial prospects of my choice of specialty?
2. Will these financial prospects meet my lifestyle expectations?

Now in Table 2, list the elements of your own vision. However, when you approximate the cost, include the emotional and time cost as well and not just the financial costs.

Remember that in the Ethics chapter of this book, I speak of Pillar 3, in which I clearly state that as humans, we are weak and make mistakes. To be balanced, we should position ourselves on the well-calibrated line that joins our ethics → choices → and our expectations. Any disturbance in this line can tilt one's balance, and this would be a recipe for collapse. Medicine is a lifestyle in which you invest all your faculties (mental, emotional, and physical), so make sure that you plan to be well aligned (your ethics → choices → and our expectations). Also, try to figure out how to be a balanced individual emotionally, intellectually, and financially. Then fill the elements of your vision with the correct timeline.

Now that you have reached the end of this chapter, you will notice that all seven steps come down to the following simple yet difficult-to-achieve notion: Understand yourself, and your choices then plan accordingly. Even when your plans do not work, use the same process to reassess your situation!

Healing: Success is from Within to Climate Creation

Hussain Isma'eel and Oussama Wazni

Successful healing is not measured by eliminating the disease. Success is a process, a climate, and an enduring outcome. Only if we as healers comprehend this will we ensure that healing is occurring. To further elaborate, let us ask ourselves the following:

1. How many residents are conscientious when treating their patients, yet we would not want to work with them?

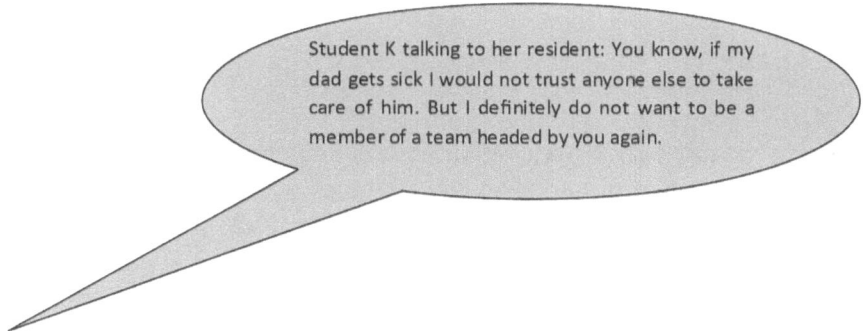

Student K talking to her resident: You know, if my dad gets sick I would not trust anyone else to take care of him. But I definitely do not want to be a member of a team headed by you again.

2. How many physicians are gifted and talented in the procedure they do, yet patients do not want to be referred to them?

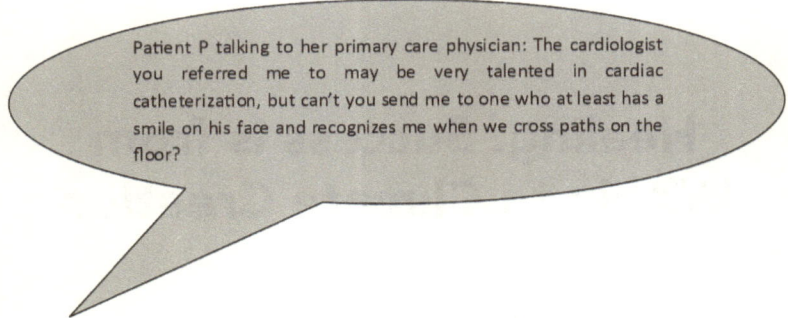

3. Is there a particular floor or ward where the environment is friendly and we wish our patients were there?

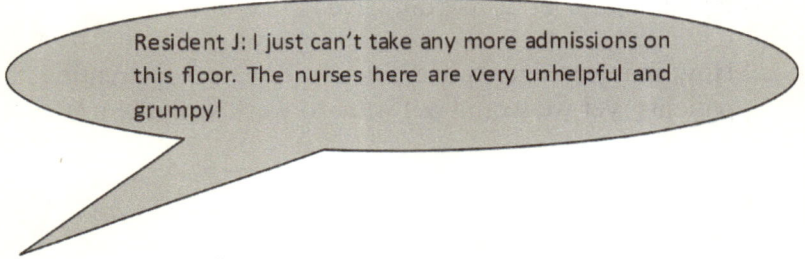

By answering the above, we have touched on what differentiates healers from practitioners. Healers are those who manage to cultivate what they are entrusted with. We are usually members of a team looking after a patient. Hence, we are entrusted with our patient's well-being and the well-being of those involved in achieving this. To cultivate means to work diligently to materialize an environment that fosters success. This environment has the following features:

a. Commitment - Each of us knows what we're supposed to do, and we trust that others will do their part also. Imagine what will happen if the lab technician forgets to calibrate the CBCD counter machine and all the results of the simple test that we routinely request are wrong. We all rely on the fact that each person is doing his/her part so we can invest our time in analyzing the data we receive instead of doubting its authenticity. Similarly, imagine what will happen if the floor intern does not order the tests while residents or consultants are waiting for a result. Behind the simplest things (CBCD), there is a process that includes a cascade of events where interruption in any of them is detrimental (see below). Communication breakdown between the teams crashes the system. The sooner we recognize that we are interconnected, the better the outcome (healing).

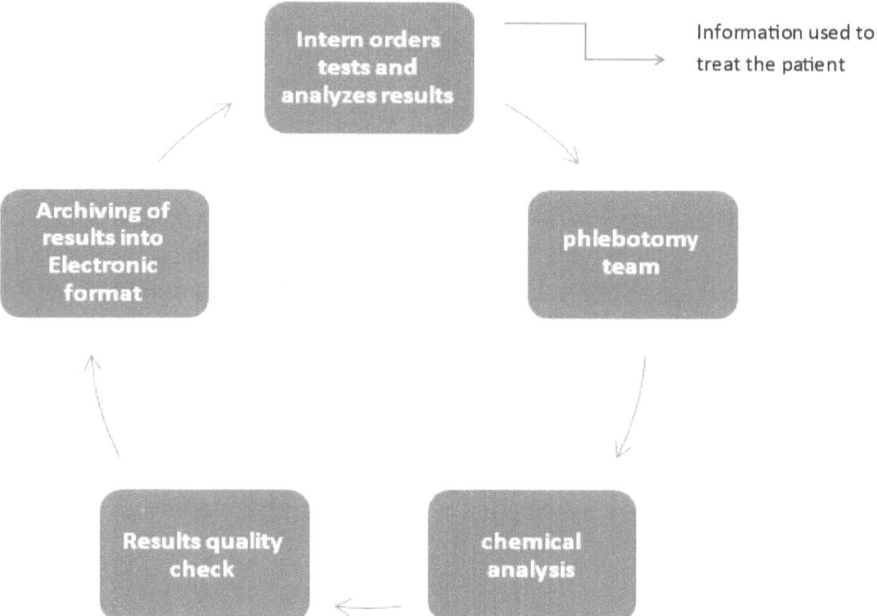

b. Optimism - Hospitals accommodate not only patients. As a matter of fact, for every patient, there are at least three other individuals servicing the patient. Therefore, if we do not make it better for each other, then this will definitely increase the negative influences in the environment of care of the patient, who is the center of this environment. Patients feel us as we feel them. Optimism is healing for patients. For students and house staff, optimism is not only looking forward to graduation, but it is also making sure that we are not unhappy in the meantime. Lack of optimism will hinder risk taking. In the chapter on outcome-based healing approach, we discovered that a fundamental part of our role is to guide our patients to take risks, ensuring that we as a team are by their side. We provide them with their prognosis after they risk a procedure. Optimism permits risk taking, and pessimism does not; both are contagious feelings.

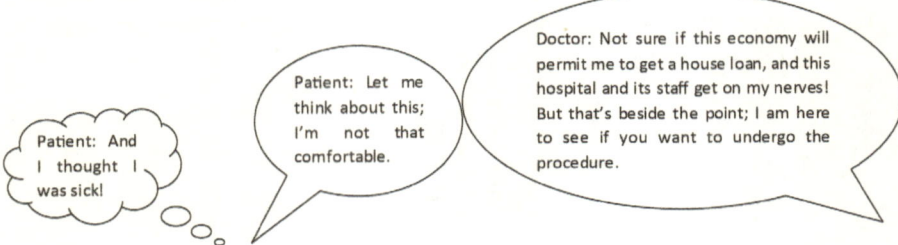

c. Collaboration - To collaborate with others, we need to know we can trust them. We need to know that they have predictably reasonable behaviors. The element of trust is essential so we know that they will do what is expected of them in our absence, similar to what they would do in our presence. Moreover, collaboration requires an understanding that unpredictable events occur, and therefore we as team members behave well facing change, i.e., we do not transmit stress onto each other. We work to de-stress a situation through focusing on problem solving with our team.

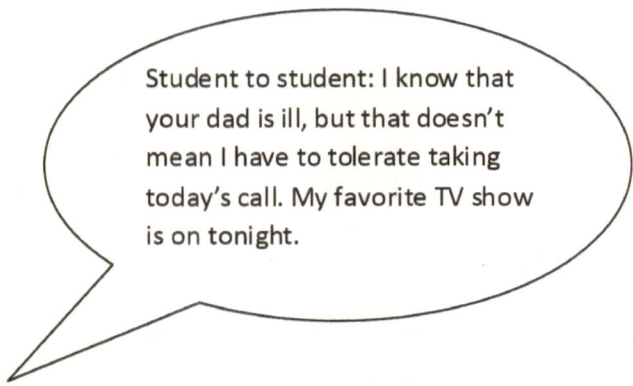

d. Accountability - One way that maturity is measured is how well a person accepts blame. In caring for patients, the situation is dynamic, i.e., it changes with time. In critically ill patients, the rate at which things change is much faster than in stable ones. Regardless of the rate of change, each patient is being attended to by a team that includes nurses, interns, residents, a primary attending physician, and consultants who are all accountable. The intern should collect all of the information from everybody, including diagnostic results and consultants' recommendations, and channel them to the resident and primary attending physician. Analyzing the results and deciding on the next steps is a joint responsibility with the rest of the team, including the resident and primary attending physician. Implementing the next steps, short of procedures, is something that the intern executes. Throughout this sequence, the intern and resident are the ones who are mostly in touch with the patient. *They are at the front line*, so they should *know* what is happening with their patients and act as those who are first to know. We should always say, "*Let me see how I can help.*" Knowledge makes them responsible. Accordingly, they should have a sense of ownership, and adopt the attitude of "*This is my patient.*" Thus, we are accountable for how we behave according to the knowledge we have with what we own. *This is our belief, attitude, and words.*

Resident at 11 am on Saturday: I wasn't on call, so I don't know why they didn't respond to the low hemoglobin level, and the student didn't inform me of this result. It wasn't me!

Versus

Resident at 11 am Saturday: I agree with you this is serious and we should have attended to our patient better. Let me first ensure we transfuse the patient now and then investigate where this problem started in my team and get back to you in 10 min.

e. Comprehensive - As we are all aware, hospitals are multilayered organizations where patient satisfaction is primary. Our patients are undergoing a multidimensional healing process. In the backstage of illness treatment, the families are struggling with securing the paperwork to ensure financial coverage of the ill individual and at the same time attending to other aspects of day-to-day life, such as jobs and the needs of other family members. From our end as healers, we should be aware that these stress factors, among others, are happening. Therefore, we should be ready to deal with the effects of these dynamics. It is not uncommon for families to displace their frustration from issues not related to the healthcare of the patient onto the system. And vice versa, it is also not uncommon that we encounter a resident or faculty who has woken up on the wrong side of the bed that day and is also displacing his or her frustrations onto the system. Neither should occur, but they do. However, our tolerance level for the patient and the family is high, while tolerance to such behavior from healers is very low. *The patient is at the center, not us!*

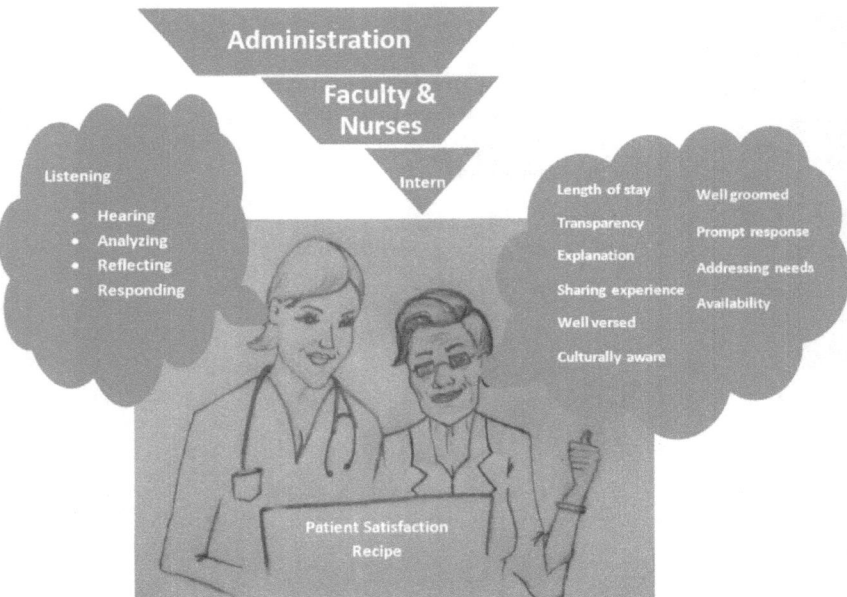

Figure by MA. Al Masri

Patients have expectations from the system at large, and we as healers are part of it, each at his/her own level. Imagine that stress like a hot bubble that expands to press on different layers all around. Each layer is separated by a spring from the other one. This spring cushions the stress and ensures that no damage occurs. We must be aware which of the patient's expectation was not met so the party responsible for that is held accountable and attends to it. Was it the length of stay? Was it the availability of the nurses, interns, or physicians? *In one of the discussions with some medical students, the following comment was made: If I were a patient and the medical practitioner in front of me is untidy and not well groomed, then this indicates he cannot take care of himself, so how can I trust him to take care of me?* This is part of what patients and their families see.

None of the above could be achieved without properly listening to the patient. Listening is an active process beyond hearing. Take a moment and ask yourself, "How can I help this individual?" Even better, ask the patient directly, "How can I help you sir/ma'am?" In the majority of the situations, the patient already has the answer; we might not need to think a lot.

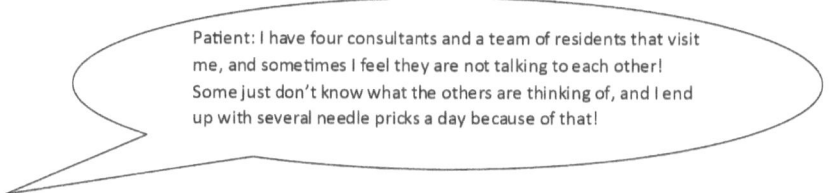

Going back to the first paragraph, healers cultivate an environment and climate that fosters success. Failure to do so can be ascribed to many reasons. However, with the right set of beliefs, commensurate attitude, and aligned behaviors, we are bound to head toward our goal. We as healers will progress during our training years to play various roles from students to senior house staff to consultants. The skills needed to perform these roles span more than reading and memorizing the gene associated with the illness. In the earlier stages, we are mostly led; later, we will be mostly leading. Moving from one role to another and mastering these roles is a process.

With this, we end this chapter and ask you to reflect on the fable below while thinking to yourself, *"I am this leader, where does this apply to me?"*

A recipe for healing leaders: the builders of this world

There was once this king, and a powerful and kind-hearted one he was. Like all the firsts of their kind, he knew exactly what he did not want to be, and less of what, and lesser of the process of how to be. However, his illusion, the shadow of his "I" on earth, showed him this order in reverse. After the thrill of achieving the throne, the vision of the projected self was observed. The pillars of the kingdom were to be raised with the labors of the lieutenants to rise. In rising, they were to claim their place, hence competing with other lieutenants, some of who are actually in guise. The force of change was in a will battle against the false fear of demise. Naturally, change was the less popular option, as stagnation is always sold by the more popular. Conversely though, not every change is for the better despite the fact that a station stinks from stagnation. Nevertheless, the leader's ship sailed in a promising wind.

From that wind, the leader inspired his crew and cabinet of the days to come. These days were to be gained by the wind, and others were to be not lost to the sea. This was the equation that determined the pace; it was powered by the wind added to the will of the crew. Similar to the effect of the good speed of reform, the momentum was to carry the leader during the years before the storm. However, trusting the wind and the water was not wise from the son of the clay, for the wind's duty is to expedite the water mill's return, save for the days when no return is to come. Hence, letting go of his anchors to gain more speed, he exposed himself to the disconnection from the clay at the bottom of the sea. Thereafter, the trip's fate was set, and what remained was for the crew to act their roles along with the members of the cabinet.

For completion, there was the wind, the ship, and the sea, and within all these, there was the crew, the cabinet, and the leader. Within the latter group of people, there were their fears, doubts, will, ignorance, knowledge, and desires. Some of the latter were in turn the doorways to the "I" of this group. And behind this "I" is "It," cunningly and deceitfully scheming for "I" to trip. And to trip is to start with a tongue slip. This slip is a gap between what is precise and accurate on one hand, and what is wishful and inaccurate on the other. This slip is to surrender to anger or to poison reason's honey by verbal display of wrangling power. This slip is to delay God's remembrance for the love of good doing. This slip is to deny the presence of ill thoughts based on absence of direct ill action, when the truth is that a plot is but a delayed or displaced ill action. This slip is to deny admitting false judgment because of fear of judgment. This slip is many things, but in essence, it is the sum effect of the fall in the trap of forgetting about "It," your eternal enemy, whose aim is to deliver you to its mother, for it is the son of fire.

Trust fluctuated among all those on the ship with each forward blow and backward wave. This carried within the wind and the salt of the sea the rust of the world to nest within the eyes, ears, mouths, lungs, and brains of the inhabitants of the ship. Naturally, those at the upper end who had the bigger "I" became less connected to those at the lower end, those who numbered more and hence potentially have a wider view. Those at the bottom end, however, were the less informed and therefore more subject to suspension in ignorance. To the misfortune, some of the cabinet members in between had long become an imprint, a head-shaking corpse, and hence a dysfunctional channel both upward and downward. A slap to bring down the rust over the communication bridges was due, but the questions were at what price and by whom? In the game, the accelerated justice and most irreversible is that of Death, for no one was touched and was to return. More importantly, nobody is untouchable. However, more importantly, in the experiment, death is a fact and a certainty, whereas why is a question with a million answers that can range from destiny to the most deviant acts of the wicked. Hence, in the maze of answering why, time and effort are lost to come back to the wall of the truth: Death is a fact.

Feeling the pain, the leader and some of his crew resonated to the tuning fork of the inner voice of the higher world. The leader decided to shine his light on the past. This is the light of his soul that goes from him back to him, making introspection a word of truth for those honestly seeking truth. This light's beam widens and strengthens with admitting to imperfections. After all, to be aware is to accept our imperfections and that he through his words is my soul's guiding force to perfection. The more I said, "It is I the weak; it is I the vulnerable; it is I the haughty; it is I who is reaping the seeds of mistrust and alienation; it is I who had become similar to who I lead; it is I who has lusted even if not by action, but by thought; it is I who had lied, if not directly, but by spreading unfounded thought; it is I who has focused on building the concrete disfavoring the building of the culture; it is I whose words had silenced the wisdom in the close; it is I who had disregarded acknowledging others in the ship; it is I who had refrained from using the power of the good and truthful word; and with every it is I," the light widened and showed me the truth and aided me to subjugate "It," which had fooled "I."

The king extricated the entangled and transparently displayed to himself everything in his heart for it to be flat. Where slips occurred was determined, and with that, the first relief of uplifting the burden transpired. With this uplifting, he straightened his spine to raise his vision and see ahead and also to be seen. From this, a wind was generated from within to inspire and regain control over the steering wheel in this stormy sea. Subsequently, the uplifting wind of these achievements brought forward the second relief. This relief was the wind from the inspired lieutenants, those with the brave hearts, who were hailing the leader's name and filling the ship's sails. Through the decision to self-correct and self-criticize, the wheel and sail were then regained. But of far more significance, the son of clay avoided going back to the clay at the bottom of the sea by regaining his anchor to clay—self-discipline and openness for constructive criticism. For no creature is beyond questioning, and any who thinks otherwise is but a transgressor. He saw that the opposite route was making him what he did not want to be, further distant from what he wanted to be, because he ignored his leadership role of perfecting the process of how to be. "It is I, the king of my inner world and therefore responsible for my actions, it is I who knows I the best after the

Creator, and may he cover from others my imperfections. For as I am the first in the concrete world, I compete to be the first to self-criticize and correct before any other. To know myself is to know my mini-god, and this is the doorway to knowledge. At the peak of my knowledge is where I am to myself: a station. In this station, I am big and aiming to be bigger. Once in the next station, I say, I am here, returning to him continuously, and he is far bigger.

Literature in Medical Education: Living Multiple Lives

Wael Jaber

A physical limitation on the human condition is that we as humans are able to experience only the life we live. Escaping this law of nature takes an enormous effort paramount to the effort and energy needed to escape the gravitational and atmospheric forces of Earth to experience living in space and zero gravity conditions. Fortunately, once we dedicate ourselves to "living other lives," the choices and options are as varied as the number of humans who have ever lived on Earth. As physicians, we are always experiencing the anxiety of whether we can really understand the other: our patients, their families, other caregivers, and so on. These anxieties can only be attenuated by learning to observe what is behind and underneath the patient and the chief complaints. We can practice the art and science of understanding the other in the same way we practice the signs on physical exam. Yet while taking the history and doing the exam, we can go behind the evident and beneath the surface to live just for a short while with this patient in their "alien world" and experience their point of view.

In the few pages that follow, we will walk together in the "other worlds" created by various writers of fiction and while in these worlds, we will experience just for a fleeting moment worlds that are different from ours. Literature does not offer you the pathophysiology or what ails an organ or system, but rather it elucidates the ailment and triumphs of humans and societies. The pathways and energy cycles are as complicated and interesting. The diagrams of energy levels and exchanges are full of arrows and loops. At the end, every fictional experience you live will give you the chance to transcend your daily experience and cycle just for a moment in another energy loop and life.

It is only through these fictionalized lives that you will escape the narrowness of your individual condition and be exposed to the experiences of many others. You will learn that what you thought was a unique hill or valley in your human life is shared by many others and that there are other hills and valleys to experience. The richness of fictional stories allows you to acquire insights to scale your current judgment against the values and lives of others.

Physician Writers: We all do it all the time. Some take it to this level.

Anton Pavlovich Chekhov	January 29, 1860–July 15, 1904	Russian	Physician and short story writer	"Medicine is my lawful wife, and literature is my mistress."
Mikhaíl Afanasyevich Bulgakov	May 15 1891–March 10, 1940	Russian	Satire, fantasy, science fiction, and historical fiction	"Yes, man is mortal, but that would be only half the trouble. The worst of it is that he's sometimes unexpectedly mortal—there's the trick!" - *The Master and Margarita*

Khaled Hosseini	March 4, 1965	Afghan-born American citizen	Fiction	"There is only one sin, and that is theft... when you tell a lie, you steal someone's right to the truth." - *The Kite Runner*
Abraham Verghese	1955	Indian born in Ethiopia/ American citizen	Medicine and novel	"Life, too, is like that. You live it forward, but understand it backward. It is only when you stop and look to the rear that you see the corpse caught under your wheel." – *Cutting for Stone*

PHYSICIANS AS WRITERS AND WRITERS AS PHYSICIANS:

In the era of electronic medical records, it is easy to remember that our careers in medicine begin as story (history) takers and story (history) re-tellers. I can always recall my first time meeting a patient as a medical student and facing the enormous task of getting her to tell me her story, that is, what brought her to this small room to talk to a complete stranger about her ailments. I, the shy medical student, tried to find an opening question or line to put her at ease and to get her talking. Sensing my inexperience, she trained her eyes beyond me to see if a more senior person is entering the room to offer support. These are the same anxieties, albeit to a lesser degree, that every new physician or patient experiences daily. Same as a writer who searches for the opening line to captivate the future reader and give a true representation of the story, the condition, and the first act of a play, a physician struggles with this opening line in every encounter.

My first patient took the lead. A lady in her mid-60s started talking about how she recently developed severe attacks of shortness of breath and that she was there to see me for asthma. Her speech was slightly pressured, and her eyes were fixed at a point beyond me.

She told me that she saw her two local doctors who confirmed her suspicion that she has asthma. In addition, she was already using the two inhalers that her granddaughter uses for asthma. I, an untrained listener, tried to find a break in her verbal avalanche to ask the questions that I had in mind. I had a list of questions that I prepared before entering the room and which I have heard the pulmonary attending and senior residents in my first clinical rotation asking the patients over the past few weeks. My patient went on, unaware of my plans. The attacks of poor breathing occurred only during the day. She blamed the newly developed asthma on her husband who bought two tropical birds and insisted on keeping them in the kitchen where she spends most of her day. This was a eureka moment for the new medical student: a bird-related pulmonary infection mimicking asthma (Is it crypto something? My memory is failing me), but I wrote the word "crypto" in my notebook while keeping my eyes on the patient (I am getting to be good at taking history and writing it down without ignoring the patient). I managed to interrupt and ask if the asthma medications were helping. She was not sure, but she was convinced that the birds had to go. I asked if her husband was okay with giving the birds away. She replied not really, but she has never approached him about the subject. Her husband is a businessman in West Africa, and he brought the birds home as a gift from one of his clients. The birds gave him something to do while at home. A quick glimpse at my watch showed me that I was 45 minutes into the history taking, and I was still in the room, now in the quagmire of the daily activities of her husband and the birds. Someone knocked on the door; it was my senior resident reminding me that my time was almost up and that he was coming in shortly with my attending physician. I waved and asked for five more minutes, then I ushered the lady to the examination bed. A quick focused exam had not yet entered my lexicon at the time. I focused on the positive findings and listened to the lungs (they were clear). I was careful about listening to any wheezing (There was no wheezing, but I heard what I thought could have been a systolic or diastolic murmur near her heart). I could not even tell if the sound was loud or soft, because I had no reference point). I was dizzy with confusion and slightly hyperventilating on the verge of fainting in the warm room. Fortunately, the door opened, and my resident ushered me out to present the case. A quick glimpse at my notebook showed me my notes: two new birds and suspected bird-related infection "crypto-something."

Is this how the story starts for every writer? A common encounter, with a couple of mental or written notes. How do these scattered words end up as a chapter, a book, a literary success? What are the magic ingredients? They could include listening, observing, inquiring, and mostly looking beyond and beneath the apparent. The medical student was back in the attending office to present the case. His mind was clouded with a few words. A 60-something-year-old lady (What does she do in life?) was suffering new onset asthma (Is it asthma or just shortness of breath?) after her husband brought two tropical birds home from West Africa (Did she travel with him to West Africa?). She has been using her granddaughter's asthma medications (What medications? I forgot to ask the names. Why is the granddaughter living with her, or does she live with her?). She has a murmur, but her lungs were clear (Did I listen to the bases and apices of the lungs? Was the murmur left parasternal or right parasternal? Did I listen in the left axillary area? Did she have edema or just fat feet?). The well-rehearsed medical plotline of chief complaints, history and present illness, prior history, system reviews, medications review, physical exam, tests and reports, and finally a list of differential diagnoses and plan of care were all jumbled in my head and nowhere on my notepad. Yet the woman was real, and so were her story, her shortness of breath, the tropical birds, and her husband. I know they were real because I listened to her heart and she had a murmur. The "story" of this lady was written two hours later. My attending resident used his investigative skill to unmask dyspnea based only on exertion, a history of heart murmur since childhood, and a mid/late mitral systolic murmur. Mitral valve prolapse and regurgitation were discovered later on an echocardiogram, and the two tropical birds remained safe, providing the husband a daily memento of West Africa.

When did the story for this woman start? What moment in her life is the starting point for her story? Do we start from the day she was diagnosed with a murmur as a child? How do we get her to talk about that moment? Do we start with the day/month when she began to experience shortness of breath? Can she recall the exact time? We often sum up the life of a patient before the present illness with an inadequate and foolish statement: The patient was in his/her usual state of health USOH until...we decided where the story begins.

The quantum leap taken by each physician who went on to become a fiction writer looks less impressive if we consider that traditionally physicians practiced the essential tools of writing ever day; these tools are keen observation of the other and transferring the thoughts and scenes from the play of life on to paper and now to computer screens.

The story was later written after a focused and rehearsed interview with the attending physician. Linear as it may sound, she had a murmur as a child, the dyspnea started about two years before the birds landed in their house, the asthma medications never helped, and she had a systolic mitral murmur that was later confirmed to indicate mitral valve prolapse with severe regurgitation. The tropical birds were saved and lived to provide the husband with a memento of his West African paradise. Still I struggled. How do we start the story of this patient? At what moment did her story really start? Was it when she was sitting in our clinic, or was it when she was diagnosed with a murmur as a child? Should we sum up all of this at an intermediate point when she started experiencing shortness of breath? How do we get her to focus on that moment? How do we know to ignore the tropical birds and the asthmatic granddaughter? Do we just resort to the known foolish and inadequate medical dictum, "The patient was in her usual state of health USOH until she started experiencing . . ."? How mediocre is this statement that fills the chart of every patient we see, a life and many lives summed up as USOH?

The inadequacy of our medical history writing may have served as an impetus for so many physicians to gravitate toward fictional writing. Physicians are awarded a rare gift, a front seat in the theater of human tragedies and triumphs. We often choose to zoom in on the scene and focus on what interest us in the spectacle. With that, we gain intimate knowledge of the "diseased organ" and lose the epical life of every patient. The literary line of physicians who became writers is long and growing. From Chekhov to Bulgakov to the modern Khaled Hosseini and Abraham Verghese, these writers answered the same calling as doctors and fictional prodigies, the call to understand and analyze human suffering and experience, and write about it to a colleague or to the public. Medical experience tends to provide the prepared mind with a long and detached view of human life. This experience teaches the physician/writer to sharpen their observational skills and zoom in and out on the scene, the character, or the surroundings. One can also think that physicians turn to writing as a therapeutic process to flush out the post-traumatic stress ideas, a process that many warriors turn to when they return home. Doctors and healers have been immersed in stories for as long as the profession existed. They were invited to enter the physical and emotional space of people, families, and communities to observe, analyze, and heal. In contrast to traditional fictional writers, physicians had to work backwards in translating the human experience and maladies into coded sentences and words that only the "priesthood" of physicians can understand fully. Writers often take the human condition and represent it to the wide audience in clear and common imagery. The plot of a fictional novel exists in every physician-patient encounter. Listen to the background of the story. Try to rewind back just a moment from when the patient wanted to start the story, and a sea of human emotions and experiences will open for you to observe or immerse yourself into. Escape into the life of your patients/characters and see the plot develop to amuse you, educate you, and make you just a bit more human.

With long years of training and working hours, why does a physician find himself/herself with the need to write and tell a story? Is it the inadequacy of the medical narrative that they have to write many times a day an impetus to break the temporal and physical boundaries of the "medical history and present illness?" When Chekhov explored the small lives of his community with his short stories, he used his medical skills to create an anatomic description of a scene and dissect the scene, uncovering layer after layer of emotions, social webs, and human failures. Chekhov was often sincere in portraying the physician in his story (often the local village/country doctor) as full human beings with lusts, desires, moral greyness, and rare triumphs. We can sense from the pages a desire to share the stories of these villagers while using the plot to provide a space for atonement for his doctors. The doctors in all these stories are never the main characters or the healing heroes. They are just part of the fabric of the community stains, wrinkles and all. In *Ward No. 6*, the doctor starts with his traditional role of a detached healer and ends as a patient in his own ward. As a physician, you will immediately identify with the universal themes that doctors face on a daily basis irrespective of the decade, the century, or even the millennia. These daily themes in any medical profession—fear, illness, hope, suffering, courage, perseverance, and death, with the occasional miracle—are omnipresent in Chekhov's writing as well as in the writing of all physicians who chose a literary medium to explore the human condition. You will even learn ironically about managed care in a story of a rural doctor who is sent to care for a large poor community in a facility where the executive powers are in the hands of administrators. This doctor has the familiar untrained, poorly paid and corrupt support staff and superiors. In a theme that is familiar in the twenty-first century, he even receives his supply of medications from a central office that determines the source of the pharmaceuticals irrespective of their effectiveness. Another story shows us the educated doctor who knows his medical theory and pathophysiology well. This doctor accumulated a wealth of theoretical knowledge, only to fail at the basic test of providing his patients with good care due to the lack of the essential ingredient: empathy. How many of your current and future co-workers can you identify in this doctor? Instead of a centralized twentieth-century "house of God," we find in Chekhov's writing many of these houses in every village and community. We also develop a rare insight into how we as physicians are perceived by patients and their families. Isn't this insight a rare chance for a much-needed ego check and psychological therapy?

Yet we in the medical profession are in the throes of titanic forces to take away from us the current ability of doctors to write a narrative, inadequate as it may have been, and replace it with electronic medical records where the breadth of the human experience and ailments are replaced with data fields and check boxes. No more are we allowed to infuse our history with subjective phrases that portray the environment in which the illness is manifesting itself. We are now confined to a series of suggested data choices from which we can pick a symptom, a prior illness, and diagnoses. These boxes and fields reflect not the richness of the human experience but the poverty and narrow view of the "administrative" and "data management" minds. Will this transition to data fields be a kiss of death to the fountain of literary minds that emerge from the medical profession? Are the EMRs going to deprive doctors of the daily practice of writing? I see many of my fellow doctors priding themselves about no longer carrying a pen or pencil anymore. The hope is that the current "recipe-like" medical notes and electronically generated "smart phrases" will be a driving force for many doctors to escape into writing fiction and use the fictional medium to explore beyond the boundaries of EMR and provide a tool of therapeutic psychological self-healing. The unintended consequence of EMR may be more like Abraham Vergheses stepping forward and bridging the gap between doctors as healers while minimizing the pain of the EMR, transforming all of us into data entry robotic white coats. The singular life we have to live on Earth may become less fulfilling when we are transformed into data generators and miners. Thus, more of us may find more reasons to escape to reading and writing fiction, and live the many lives of other characters and physical spaces. The EMR does not allow a space for us to explore the things our patients enjoyed, currently enjoy, or want to enjoy in the future. The binary concept of "present" and "absent" required by EMR provide us a sterile and distant representation of our subjects (the patient). The EMR has no time or space for the two tropical birds or for the fact that the patient did not have a prescription but yet was taking her granddaughter's medications. Again, why does her granddaughter live with her?

Electronic Medical Records Systems: Another tool with its own value and price	
Pro	Con
1. **Readability (no handwriting clarity issues)**	1. **Decreased efficiency in launching and during learning curve phase**

2. Ability to transfer data

2. Generation of new types of errors (facilitates propagation of error through Copy/Paste)

3. Expedite translating data into different languages

3. Can lead to communication breakdown if it limits interaction with colleagues

4. Remote access for healthcare networks

4. Costly (purchasing, training, and maintenance) and needs continuous upgrading

5. Facilitate data mining (research, quality improvement, and patient safety studies)

5. Vulnerability (linked to software designer company)

6. Reduce time for data entry (create shortcuts for commonly used phrases)

6. Limited system-to-system cross talk

7. Clinical decision making support (built-in reminders, notifications for drug-drug interactions)

7. Patient's privacy issues are a continuous concern

8. Reduce error by having a computerized ordering system

8. Overdependence on technology

9. Reduce lag time from order entering by physicians to order implementation by nurses

9. Power shift within organizations

10. Improves patient safety and other clinical outcomes

10. Create a new/different type of work for physicians

11. Advantages can go beyond institutions to societal and public health levels	11. Negative emotions (if not all end users are integrated in the system, work shifting will occur and create resentment)
	12. Duplication of effort (some continue to take notes on paper before entering data)

Finally, as you enter a career of continuous learning and humbling encounters, it is healing to escape through reading fiction into a world of made-up characters where your input is not needed, the flow of the story is not your responsibility, and the angle from which human life is seen is new and wide. You will start seeing yourself and your patients in some of the characters as humans who are trying to make the best out of an unfair universe. You will revitalize your fountain of empathy from the behavior of the failing characters, or you may discover this empathy and learn to get the full story from your patients and unfocus just for a while from the chief complaints and organ-specific history taking and exam. You may start seeing your patients not as a failing elderly in this moment and time, but as humans who were once loved by a caring family, celebrated birthdays, and suffered a broken arm after climbing a tree, as individuals who were teased in middle school and fell in and out of love in their youth. These patients are parents whose young kids run to with open arms when they return from work. They are among your patients, and they are people who dreamed of and saved for a vacation. The frail elderly man in front of you may have walked his daughter down the aisle to give her away to a loving husband. Each of these patients can recount the totality of the human experience on Earth, yet they are here in front of you with a specific ailment. How inadequate are their history and present illness in reflecting their lives?

Author Biography

Like the majority of my colleagues during our learning years, we were not properly guided on making the right career decisions. Everybody would keep repeating the cliché "Do what is right for you." The challenge was to be able to formulate the elements of the vision of what is right for us. Only by knowing these elements would one be able to make the right decision. In a way, many of my colleagues, including myself, were asking for the informed consent paper so we know what career we are signing into.

With the above in mind, my track was somehow different from my peers in the fact that I was a more daring experimentalist. I did not mind taking on assignments and going through tracks with the aim of investigating and exploring myself in these paths. I thought, if you will not show me a checklist of what this field is about, then I will try it and develop my own. Naturally, this meant engaging in tracks and completing the assignments, but then moving on to try another.

This is why when the field of gene therapy was gaining momentum, I was under the impression that this modality will be at the bedside within few years and I need to really know how this is going to revolutionize the field. At the Massachusetts General Hospital, I was introduced to this field by Prof. Xandra Breakefield and Prof. Richard Masland. We sought to cure blindness by introducing genes with the herpes simplex virus. We received a high score on our R21 grant and in the words of Dick, this was my welcome sign from the capitalist world. Later, they both taught me patience, and this experience disillusioned me about gene therapy. Having moved back to clinical medicine at AUB, Prof. Samir Alam (cardiology), Prof. Kamal Badr (nephrology), and Prof. Ali Taher (hematology) made sure I remain engaged in research and work at the overlap areas between cardiology and the other two fields. Clinical research started to look different, and with Ali Taher, the cardiovascular complications of Thalassemia proved a very educationally enlightening track. Later on, the late Prof. Munir Shamaa (gastroenterology), with whom I used to discuss my writings and also treat as a patient, was approached by Ms. Amal Saeed to help solve my predicament and was the person who said, *"Money should not stop someone like you. I want to give you this 5000 USD check knowing that it is not enough for a full scholarship, but it will get you at the doorstep. This is how I got to Boston in the 1950s; I wiped the floors of the ship, and I am sure you will make it."* Prof. Samir Alam generously ensured that the rest is covered. He was not about to let one of his favorite students fail to reach the next stage. He believed this was part of his mentorship. At Harbor-UCLA, Prof. Matthew Budoff showed me the world of cardiac imaging and specifically cardiac CT in a different way. His passion, belief in the modality, and relentless efforts to train, publish, and do what it takes to promote cardiac CT were contagious. Thereafter, starting my career as director of Cardiac Imaging at Beirut Cardiac Institute was not a simple undertaking. With Dr. Mohammad Saab and Dr. Mohammad Bachir, I learned what it means to answer the questions the cardiac surgeon needs to ensure the best outcome and what it means to operate in a startup project and keep the ship financially and administratively sober, respectively. Missing research and contemplating a wider impact, I moved back to AUB as codirector of the Vascular Medicine Program. Along with my colleagues from engineering, nutrition, public health, clinical chemistry, and healthcare administration, we led intra-hospital and national initiatives. We were set to address our local challenges. Our investments had to be in creating infrastructure, capacity building, and in areas that impact our clinical practice. If whatever we investigated or studied cannot be implemented, then it was not a priority.

Abiding to the principle of coupling research to implementation, as a group we launched the salt reduction program, called the Lebanese Action on Salt and Health (LASH); the Women Heart Health Center, a center dedicated to providing outpatient preventive cardiology care free of charge for underprivileged women; the BisPhenol A and Cardiovascular Health Working Group; the Greater Beirut Area Cardiovascular Cohort (GBACC) to study the relationship between dietary factors, genetic factors and cardiovascular diseases, and outcomes; and the CARE Program, an electronic record-based program to implement quality of care improvements within the participating network of hospitals. None of these programs could have come to existence without the wonderful prevailing team spirit of the individuals involved in them. Mr. Mohammad Medawar stands out as the talented research assistant who we could depend on and delegate to, knowing things will be accomplished effectively and efficiently.

For some external observers, including some trusted friends, this change in paths did not reflect well on me. At some point of time, it actually got to me, and I asked myself and trusted seniors in the field how it is that many of the people I work with focus on a single track, while I am very close to being described as all over the map.

To answer the above question, we approached it from two angles: How productive was I in comparison to the focused group, and what is the origin of this pattern? From the productivity standpoint that was answered by a revered and more established figure who eventually stated this is that probably just who I am. As for the origin of this pattern, that was up to me to figure out. I found the following answers: I am in the searching period, and it happens that I was more willing to give this more time than others; since a lot of my decisions were not purely dictated by career issues (financial constraints), then my approach was realistic and matched my needs; and the role models I looked up to were scientists/philosophers such as Avicenna and Descartes. The latter reason is actually at the core of why I was so daring. From my readings and understanding of these icons, I saw in them individuals who were always capable of bridging the conceptual to the concrete. They functioned as implementation channels— very prolific channels. In their own worlds, they conceptualized, experimented, and then refined their conceptual framework. In my simplistic terms, they wrote a checklist of what something is all about. To them, mastering the scientific methodology enables you to project it in various fields.

With this background, this book was written with the intent to provide medical students a collected version of what this medical career is about. They are introduced to the conclusions drawn from the abovementioned experiences. This is a guide that focuses on the "how" to do and is balanced by presenting the conceptual background of this "how." Keeping in mind that this guide had to be compact and should serve as an introduction to the readers for them to formulate their own idea, I request each reader to take the time to criticize any gaps, add to it, and someday write his/her own further developed version. Every experience is unique in its concrete shape.

Book Description

"Why did you write this book?" I was asked by friends. My answer was, "I wanted to put what you have taught me and how it was further shaped by experience in a way not told before. It will speak our minds. It will document it so we become known and have not departed without having registered how we think the practice of medicine ought to be." This guide needs to target the medical students we are teaching, for the journey starts there. They have to be properly guided in their career and better introduced to the "how'" of becoming healers. It is about time the collective wisdom that we all acquire with experience and time, which shows us that many of our choices could have been better had we been better coached, is documented. This collective wisdom is that which speaks many truths, and of which the following are among its leading statements: Do not settle for what is just not bad, for under stress that might become bad; perfecting the act is an added value per se; the smart learn from their mistakes, but the wise learn from others' mistakes; blessed are those who know where they are, where they were, and where they are heading; a practicing learned physician is in his acts acting out of benevolence; remember that fairness is in equity not equality; and whatever you wish that men would do to you, do so to them.

At first glance, the medical student reading the above might question how this applies to him/her. It is this guide's duty to address this question. As noted in the book's summary, this guide is composed of seven chapters that aim to uncover some processes of how to become medical healers. It was written to include a conceptual framework, a step-by-step guide to the process, exercises, and real stories and reflections to further help clarify the implementation aspect of the guide. The scope of this book starts from a historical background that reveals some of the dynamics that continue to exist in the minds of people about physicians. Then, the guide details the thinking process that leads to forming a differential diagnosis and how to practice in an outcome-based manner. Furthermore, this book provides suggestions on how students should choose their subspecialty and introduces them to basic fundamental concepts about patient satisfaction. There is one overarching spirit prevailing over this guide, and that is the universality of ethical principles of practice.

In further details, we as medical physicians join the medical track with several preconceived ideas in our head. How many of these ideas actually remain after we graduate and how many remain after we practice for a number of years are two different questions. If the ideas we joined the field for are not those that are really part of the practice, then we were under some kind of an illusion. Here, it is worth noting a reality that is not widely promoted, which is that the medical degree is not only a license to diagnose diseases and prescribe medications; it is far much more than that. Yes, graduates with a medical degree are expected to be treating physicians. However, many of them do not become so. Those who become clinicians come to learn that it takes more than the medical knowledge we acquired in medical science books to become a successful clinician. Institutions that have understood that provide their house staff and faculty with courses on communication skills, conflict resolution, inclusiveness, and professionalism. The Cleveland Clinic, which is the number one heart care facility in the USA, is a living example of such institutions. The Clinic has clearly set the patient as the top priority, and recognizing that human–human interaction is a bi-directional relationship, the Cleveland Clinic ensures that their end of the interaction is well prepared. In this guide, the section that discusses patient satisfaction provides clear examples of what team spirit is in implementation. Furthermore, this section highlights that this is a climate that ensures everybody's success. Individualism in its negative facets will not take a clinician far. Creating a climate of success entails that it is a continuous process in which medical students and house staff play a pivotal role. This category is at the front desk of our institutions relative to the patient and therefore, they need to be well prepared.

Other sections explain statistical concepts such as understanding posttest probabilities and disease pattern recognition. However, this guide presents these ideas in what we believe is a more integrated manner. We aimed to avoid presenting this material in a fragmented way that replicates some of the dry stat courses we attended. Instead, we wanted to link the logic of clinical decision making to statistics and then to what and how we communicate our messages to the patient, and to what needs to be monitored and documented in the progress note. Linking all these together was not a simple undertaking, and this is because this is how it is in reality. In fact, any medical student should recognize earlier on that the experience of healing a patient is a single interaction. It is only for research and educational purposes that we separate the elements of this healing process into history and physical exam, statistics, pathophysiology, imaging and lab testing, and message communication. In other words, the separation is an artifact created by the medical schools to facilitate teaching us. However, later on, we should put all the parts of the puzzle together to see the healing experience as a complete entity.

In terms of disease recognition and differential diagnosis formation, this guide acknowledges a facet of this challenge upfront. This feature is that during the theoretical knowledge acquisition years (Med 1 and 2 in the American system), students are taught the name of the disease, what causes it, how it manifests, and then the treatment and course of healing. After these two years and in our clinical practice, we are operating somehow in reverse, as we start by collecting features to form patterns that may be caused by a set of diseases (called a differential set) and then try to work our way to identify the true disease. This "walk in reverse" is not a simple switch to be understood and perfected by many. It takes time and is a craft. We tried to simplify this by introducing methodological processes that are generic and once practiced can help in forming a differential diagnosis for all complaints.

Furthermore, many times early in our careers, and given that time is precious and we are pressured to decide on what path are we going to follow, we tend to anchor ourselves to wrongly formed first impressions about certain specialties. The section that provides suggestions about how to choose a specialty aims in its gist to help the medical student discern the true facet of the specialty in general from what is particular to how this specialty is practiced at this institution by these faculty members in particular. Only by doing so will medical students be able to know what they are subscribing to as long- term careers and not find what they learned about the nonmedical aspects of the specialty being practiced in a very different way in other places.

Finally, we who adopt the methodologies highlighted in this guide are committed, faithful believers in the universality of humans and their thoughts. No overarching principle is new under this sun. All have been present since the beginning, and it's up to us to discover these principles. Of these principles are the principles of ethical practice of medicine. They can be traced back to the Hindu Vaidya's oath of medical practice in 1600 BC to Chinese Taoism and Confucianism to Assaf's oath in the Jewish heritage, to the Hippocratic oath, to the teachings of Jesus Christ, to the teachings of Islam, and to the United Nations Human Rights Declaration. However, while ethical principles are universal, it is their application that differs, and respecting variations in their application is part of adhering to them. Otherwise, how can we admire autonomy and respect toward others (as in patients) and not be willing to do the same to fellow physicians from other cultures? This in brief is what this guide describes and what it is about. We truly hope that students will find in it answers to some of their questions and assist them to become the healers we aspire for them to be.

www.ingramcontent.com/pod-product-compliance
Lightning Source LLC
Chambersburg PA
CBHW030751180526
45163CB00003B/984